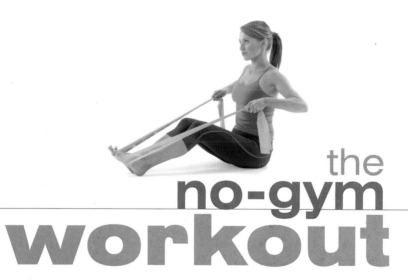

the
no-gym
workout

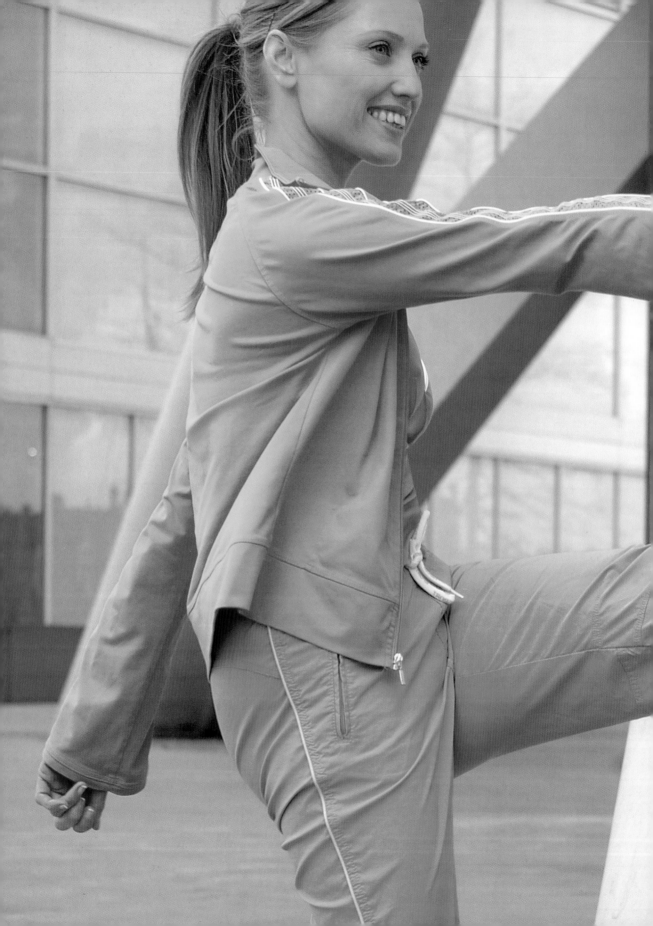

RODALE

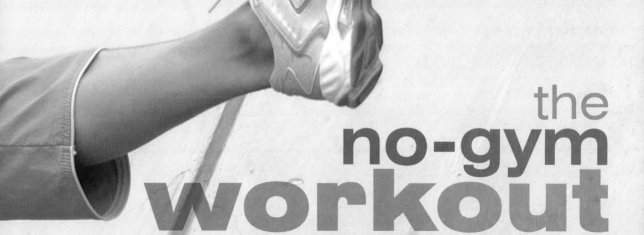

the
no-gym
workout

Tone up, burn fat, lose inches – in just 6 weeks

Lucy Wyndham-Read

This edition first published in the UK in 2007 by
Rodale International Ltd
7–10 Chandos Street
London W1G 9AD
www.rodalebooks.co.uk

Printed and bound by Star Standard Industries (PTE), Singapore, using
acid-free paper from sustainable sources.

1 3 5 7 9 8 6 4 2

A CIP record for this book is available from the British Library
ISBN-13: 978-1-4050-9984-4

Contributing writer Liz Dean
Art direction and design Hannah Moore
Project editor Angela Baynham
Senior editor Liz Coghill
Managing editor Anne Lawrance
Photographer Mike Prior
Illustrator Kevin Smith
DTP Keith Bambury
Production controller Sara Granger

This paperback edition distributed to the book trade by
Pan Macmillan Ltd

Notice

The information in this book is meant to supplement, not replace, proper exercise
training. All forms of exercise pose some inherent risks. The editor and publisher
advise readers to take full responsibility for their safety and know their limits. Before
practising the exercises in this book, be sure that your equipment is well maintained,
and do not take risks beyond your level of experience, aptitude, training and
fitness. The exercise programme in this book is not intended as a substitute for any
exercise routine that may have been prescribed by your doctor. As with all exercise
programmes, you should get your doctor's approval before beginning.
Mention of specific companies, organisations or authorities in this book does
not imply endorsement by the publisher, nor does mention of specific companies,
organisations or authorities in the book imply that they endorse the book.
Websites and telephone numbers given in this book were accurate at the time
the book went to press.

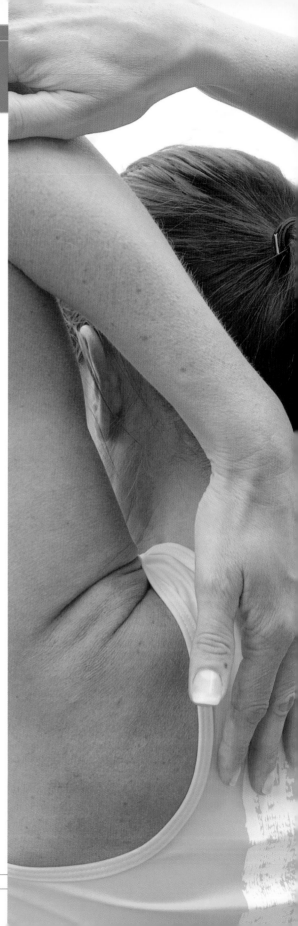

contents

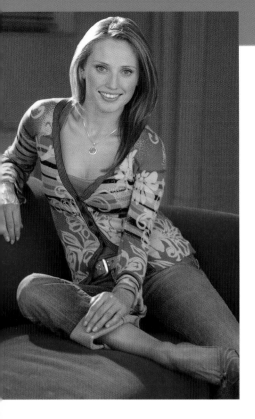

introduction

A couple of years ago, I was working out at a local gym I'd recently joined. I noticed it was really quiet – although it was early evening, only two or three of us were using the facilities. Sitting on the exercise bike I stopped for a minute to take a look around me. I counted about 20 pieces of cardio equipment and 10 fixed weight machines, one for each muscle group. I asked the gym manager, 'How many members does the gym have?'

'Eighteen hundred,' he replied.

'But,' I queried, 'you have only 10 fixed weight machines and 20 pieces of cardiovascular equipment. What are you going to do when all the members turn up? There won't be enough machines to go round.'

'Oh,' he replied, confidently, 'they won't come.'

That conversation prompted me to write this book. Leisure organisations are well aware that people who join a gym often quickly stop going because they get bored and their workout takes too long. There are lots of us who pay the sign-up fee, then the monthly membership – but rarely go often enough to justify this commitment. We might feel guilty about spending the money, yet few of us turn up enough times to get value for money out of our membership. Regardless, we remain gym members because we want to hold onto the idea that we're committed to our health and to fitness. We feel that giving up the membership would mean that we would somehow be giving up on getting fit. But it doesn't have to be that way – stopping wasting money on a gym you don't go to is your first step towards regaining control of your life and, with the help of this book, getting the figure you want on your own terms.

There are lots of reasons why many people have never joined a gym: because they have young children to look after, they have demanding jobs, they travel a lot, they can't afford the fees or they just don't feel comfortable in a gym environment. I have written the No-Gym Workout for all those people as well as for those who are paying for membership but not using it. I want to prove that you don't need a gym or specialist equipment to get fit, tone up and feel good about your body – a good pair of trainers and an exercise mat are the only really essential items you need to get started on the programme. Just follow the toning exercises (at home or at work), enjoy the power walks and eat healthily, and you'll see great results in just six weeks.

how will this workout save me time?

The No-Gym Workout involves doing three toning exercises three times each week, plus power walks. The exercises are designed to take less time than an equivalent workout in the gym, yet tone the same number of muscles.

I'll give you an example. At my local gym, I watched a new member, exercise card in hand, work her way through her exercise programme. She began on the chest-press machine, then moved onto the tricep extension machine, and finally onto an exercise mat to do sit-ups – but to achieve the same results all she needed to do were press-ups. The box press-up in Week 01 (see page 48) uses exactly the same muscles as two machines and the sit-ups, and consequently takes only a third of the time to do. This is how the No-Gym Workout maximises your use of the precious time you have, but doesn't compromise on getting you fit. Each move works intensively, toning one or more muscle groups together.

You'll also enjoy the flexibility of this programme – the beauty of it is that you can do any of the three exercises at any time of day you choose. You might like to fit in the upper-body exercise after breakfast, do a middle-body exercise, such as the ab rolls, after work or while you're watching television, and the lower-body exercise, such as a leg kick, while you're waiting for the kettle to boil. This means that you'll always be able to find the time to work out – see how my case study clients managed to fit their workout around their lifestyles on pages 54, 66, 78, 90, 102 and 114.

'The No-Gym Workout maximises your use of the precious time you have, but doesn't compromise on getting you fit.'

getting motivated

I love a challenge, which is probably why I joined the army. I learned a lot about working with people and about what motivates others to excel themselves. In five years I crawled through tunnels, trekked for miles in thunderstorms, and pushed myself to the limit. It wasn't easy, but because of these experiences I know how fantastic it feels to achieve something you once thought impossible – and also, how it feels to fail, to lose motivation and to slip backwards rather than make real progress.

Motivation is essential. We all know that exercise and healthy eating are good – but why is it so hard to put them into practice consistently? How do you keep going into week 2, week 3, week 4, when the novelty of the new diet and exercise regime has worn off? This book is packed with ways to stay motivated,

'I know from experience that when my clients do exercises and power walking that they enjoy, they succeed – they get the body they want without going anywhere near a gym.'

from setting realistic goals to rewarding yourself for your success. It deals with the emotional patterns that can inspire or diminish your chances of success, and helps you enjoy the process of getting a stronger, leaner body. I know from experience that when my clients do exercises and power walking that they enjoy, they succeed – they get the body they want without going anywhere near a gym.

why it's for everyone

This programme is designed to get everyone fit, regardless of how old you are or what level of fitness you are starting from. Every exercise has an advanced version – boost the burn – so you can always challenge yourself a little more as you work through the six-week programme. You can mix and match the exercises, too, to create your own maintenance programme after the six weeks (see pages 134–5), plus there's a postnatal workout (see pages 126–33) and recommendations for workouts according to your body shape. Whether you're an apple, pear or runner bean, you can adapt the programme to your needs and enhance your figure.

in this book

You will find ways to motivate yourself.
You will find the exercises you need to tone up, lose weight and look great.
You will get the information you need to work on your body shape, whether you're postnatal or battling with your natural shape – pear, apple or runner bean.
You will see the results other women have achieved.
Your questions about the programme will be answered (see the Q&As on pages 55, 67, 79, 91, 103 and 115).
You will understand how exercising helps sleep, bones, stress levels, heart, breathing and skin (see the features on pages 56, 68, 80, 92, 104 and 116).
You will get off a negative spiral and into a positive mindset.
You will find the support you need to get healthy and slim for life.

Whatever your age, size or attitude, may you achieve your goals and enjoy the feeling of vitality and confidence that comes naturally with better health.

Lucy Wyndham-Read

Lucy Wyndham-Read   *www.lucywyndhamread.com*

wills and won'ts on the No-Gym Workout

You **will** feel fantastic

You **will** enjoy shopping for new clothes

You **will** love getting ready to go out in the evenings

You **will** feel more energised morning and night

You **will** thrive on compliments

You **will** feel more attractive

You **will** feel and look years younger

You **will** improve your posture

You **will** feel stronger and fitter

You **won't** waste money on a gym membership

You **won't** have yo-yo weight problems

You **won't** feel out of breath when you walk up the stairs

You **won't** miss the clothes you've slimmed out of

You **won't** have to ask, 'Does my bum look big in this?'

You **won't** feel guilty about an occasional dessert

You **won't** envy celebrity bodies – because you'll be happier with yours

You **won't** feel your weight is out of control

You **won't** have a single excuse not to exercise

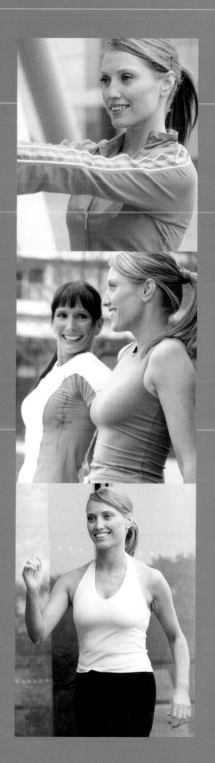

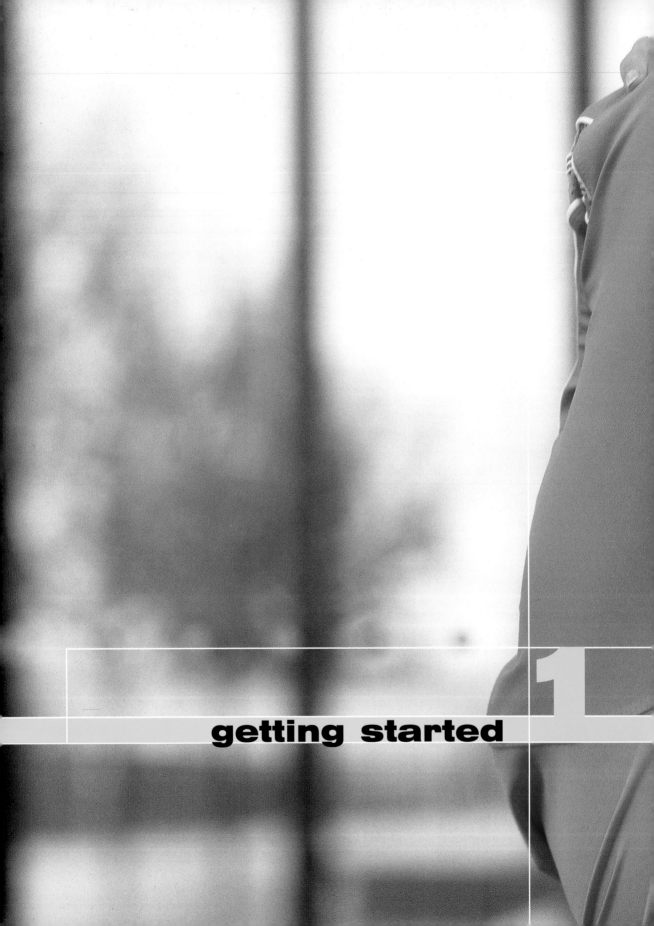

getting started

1

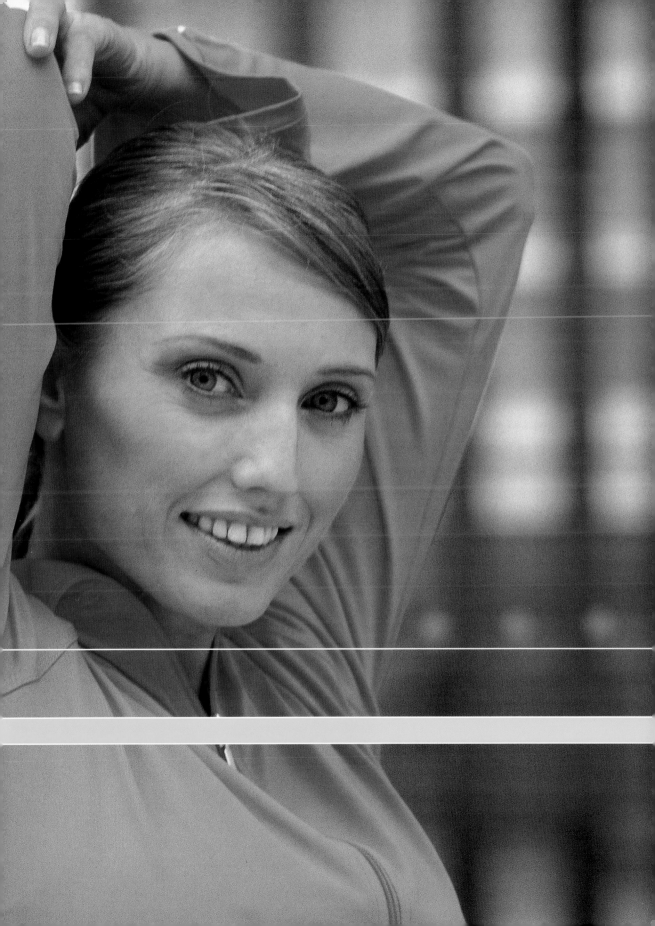

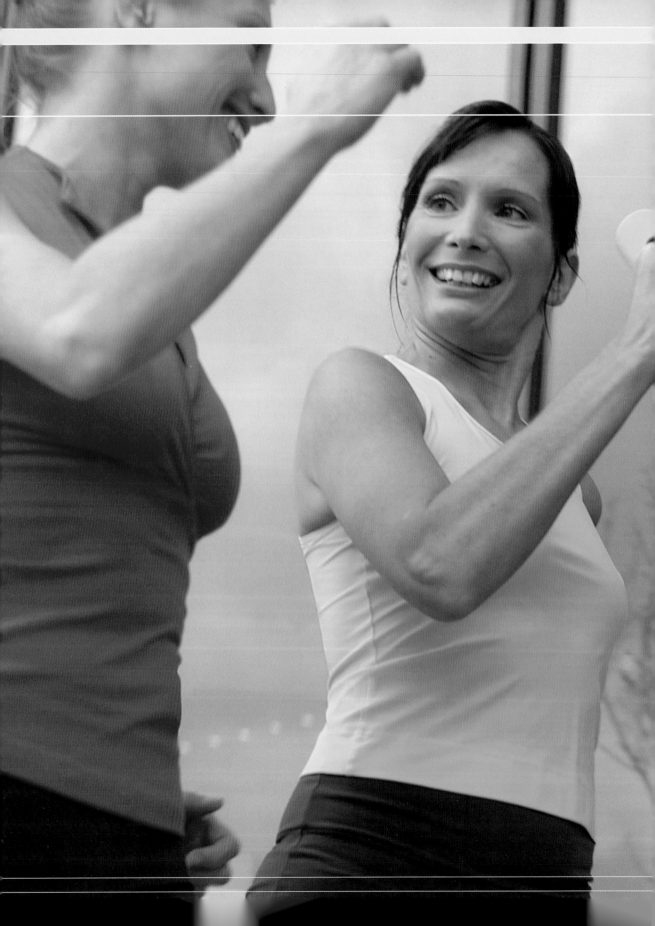

burn it off!

the metabolic miracle
for inch loss

You don't need to take drastic action for a miracle
to happen. All you do need to do is tone one day to raise
your metabolism, then power walk the next to burn off
body fat. Walking is the most natural form of exercise
there is, toning every muscle while burning the highest
number of calories. By adopting this specially created
exercise programme you will notice the changes in your
figure as well as in the way you feel in a matter of weeks.
And you can spend the money the No-Gym Workout saves
you on gym membership on a well-earned healthy treat at
the end of the six weeks.

raising your metabolism
the principle of the programme

Many people blame their inability to reduce their size on the fact that they have a naturally slow metabolism. However, the idea that metabolic rate is fixed is pure fiction – a slow rate is generally due to low fitness levels often caused by a sedentary lifestyle. In fact, you can raise your metabolic rate and increase your calorie-burning potential at will. Simply work through the programme and kickstart your metabolism.

what is your metabolic rate?

Metabolism is a Greek word, meaning change or transformation. Metabolism is the process by which your body transforms food, internal muscle and fat into available energy. The basal metabolic rate (bmr), or resting metabolic rate, is the minimum number of calories your body needs to function while at rest. Up to 70 per cent of your daily intake of calories is burned up by the basal metabolism. It therefore follows that by revving up your metabolism, you can raise your bmr and dramatically increase your calorie-burning potential while you're resting.

HOW TO CALCULATE YOUR METABOLIC RATE

You can calculate your approximate metabolic rate using this formula:

**Your basal = your body weight
metabolic rate in pounds x 10Kcal**

Example: Multiplying your weight of, say, 150lb (67.5kg) by 10Kcal gives a metabolic rate of 1500. This means you naturally burn around 1500 calories a day without being active. This calculation is a general guide only, as it does not factor in those people who are very athletic, with a high proportion of lean muscle, or those who are very overweight.

Various factors impact on your bmr. For example, as you age your bmr drops (see pages 16–17). The weather also has an effect because you burn more calories keeping warm in cold weather and keeping cool in hot weather.

why tone and walk?

Muscle tone plays a key role in determining your metabolic rate and your body's ability to burn off calories. Muscle is the most metabolically active part of your body, and it burns up to three times more calories than any other tissue – each 450g (1lb) of muscle burns a massive 70 calories a day at rest, whereas each 450g (1lb) of fat burns only 2 calories a day at rest.

Toning exercises create lean muscle, and the more lean muscle you have, the more calories your body burns. So toning up increases your metabolic rate and helps your body burn more calories throughout the day.

Included for each toning exercise in the No-Gym Workout (see Chapter 2) is the number of calories burned once you have completed all the repetitions for the basic exercise. If you increase the intensity, you will burn off even more. These figures were calculated by asking our six case studies to do each of the exercises wearing a special wrist watch to measure the calories burned. An average of the totals gave the final count. The figures given are approximate, as individual calorie-burning potential depends on muscle mass and other lifestyle factors, but they will give you a guide.

In addition to the toning exercises, the No-Gym Workout requires you to power walk three or four times a week (see pages 34–5). Power walking also helps you to tone up, but principally this exercise burns fat – so the combination of power walking and toning melts fat, tones muscles and ultimately gets you in shape in six weeks.

eat and drink

Your eating patterns influence your metabolism, so making key changes to what and when you eat will help you lose weight (see pages 20–3). Regular, balanced eating is the key to keeping your metabolism revved up, and you don't need to cut out the carbs, either. A healthy, balanced diet will help you support your body as you work through the No-Gym Workout.

Drinking eight or more glasses of water a day (see page 23) will ensure that your muscles perform at their peak, as well as keeping your body hydrated and enhancing your overall sense of wellbeing. Make sure you have water close at hand whenever you are exercising.

FACT

Toning exercises help you feel and look younger for longer. Your metabolic rate naturally slows down by 2 per cent for every decade of your life, but regular toning exercises halt this and help you to maintain a higher metabolic rate (see pages 16–17). Regular weight-bearing exercises also help to maintain bone density and prevent the onset of osteoporosis caused by hormonal changes during menopause.

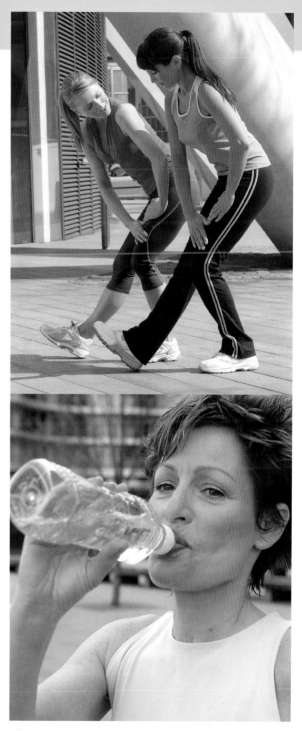

Always warm up your muscles *before embarking on any form of exercise (top).* ***Drink plenty of water*** *before, during and after exercise to keep your body hydrated (above).*

metabolism and age
exercise for the time of your life

The reason you may find it harder to lose weight as you get older is down to changes in your basal metabolic rate (bmr). This drops by 2 per cent for every decade of your life. Also, you lose 3.2kg (7lb) of lean body mass with every decade, which is replaced by fat. Therefore, as you get older you need to change what you do to stay fit, slim and toned – you need to do more exercise to turn back the clock.

You probably think that you exercise enough and, aside from the odd comfort-food snack, your diet is reasonably healthy. But deep down, you know that things simply aren't what they used to be. You can't lose weight quite so easily as you once could (although you've put your mind to it often enough) and now even minor food offences incur a hefty penalty as your thighs appear to expand in mere anticipation of a low-fat muffin.

While we may be able to hide growing curves and a burgeoning discomfort during the darker winter months, there comes an inevitable time when the protests of too-tight jeans cutting into waists and tortuous short-sleeved tops clinging to podgier arms cannot be ignored. When your wardrobe turns rebellious, it's time to find the underlying cause and take action before you lose motivation and self-esteem.

Every decade of your life presents new and varied health challenges and benefits. You may feel you were at your physical best in your twenties, but at that point you lacked the self-assurance you went on to enjoy in your thirties. In your forties, you may feel you are growing in confidence and fully accepting who you are, but then thyroid problems may arise, along with the journey towards menopause. Throughout all these life phases, your metabolism slows – but with regular exercise, you can compensate for the shift. Here's an overview of what happens to your metabolism throughout your life phases.

metabolism by the decade

in your twenties In your early twenties you naturally have more lean muscle and less fat, so your metabolic rate will be high. By your mid-twenties, if you're not exercising regularly – concentrated exercise, such as power walking, cycling or aerobics, say three times a week – muscle mass starts to decline. The muscle fibres de-activate, which slows down the basal metabolic rate, and the body's fat stores increase. However, staying in shape in your twenties can be easier than in your thirties or forties as you're more likely to have an active life with time available to spend on yourself.

in your thirties The thirties can be a time of plateau in terms of body shape and self-attitude, as we become absorbed with children, home, career development – or all three. You may feel extraordinarily busy, but don't seem to be able to shape up as you naturally lose lean muscle and gain fat.

Extra weight tends to head for the hips on women, and we often try to run it all off or we focus purely on any exercise that gets our bottoms moving in the hope of shifting weight. What's really needed, however, is toning exercises – not only because toning helps you to control your shape, but crucially because toning also helps to protect against osteoporosis (see pages 68–9). Begin (or continue) the programme during your thirties, and your body will be radically stronger by the time you reach your fifties.

in your forties During your forties, your bmr and digestive system start to slow down. Hormone fluctuation can arise at this time, particularly in the mid to late forties with the onset of menopause; again, bone density can be improved with regular toning exercises helping to prevent osteoporosis.

In addition, thyroid problems are more likely to arise during this decade. The thyroid gland in the neck helps to regulate the bmr. When it is not functioning properly, weight, energy levels, muscle strength, skin, hair and periods are affected. Too much thyroxine (the hormone produced by the thyroid) in the body can cause thyrotoxicosis, doubling the bmr. Too little thyroxine results in myxoedema, when the bmr may drop to 30–40 per cent below its normal rate. Because exercise speeds up the metabolic rate, it's helpful for those with an underactive thyroid.

in your fifties The average age for the onset of menopause is 51. During the menopause the body produces less oestrogen, which can cause the rapid loss of bone density. For some women, the hormonal changes can trigger weight gain. Given that the metabolic rate continues to slow with age unless it's speeded up by regular exercise, menopause weight gain can be difficult to lose.

in your sixties and beyond During the sixties, weight generally returns to normal. This is also a time when cholesterol levels need monitoring to protect the health of your heart. There are three types of cholesterol, or fats, in the body (see page 92): LDL (low-density lipoprotein), HDL (high-density lipoprotein) and VLDL (very low-density lipoprotein). The ratio between them indicates whether or not excess cholesterol is being deposited in the artery walls, increasing the risk of heart disease and stroke. Aerobic exercise helps to decrease LDL cholesterol and raise HDL, as can eating fewer saturated fats (see page 21).

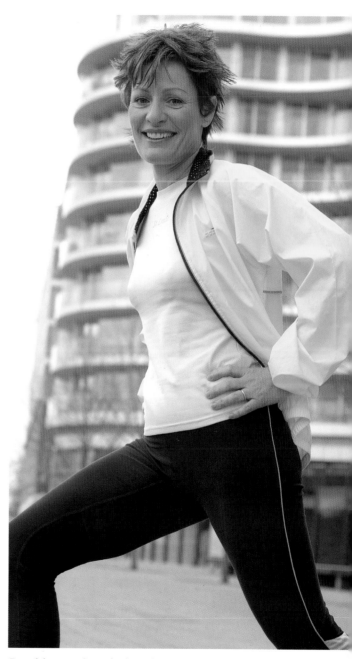

Exercising consistently throughout your life helps to protect you against conditions such as osteoporosis (loss of bone density), which can affect post-menopausal women.

under the skin
muscle know-how

The exercises in this programme use each of the six major muscle groups: chest, back, abdominals, thighs, buttocks and arms. Many are compound exercises, which means you use multiple muscles during the same exercise, with two or more joints in movement. Your body needs even muscle toning, and compound exercises give it a balanced programme that works all the major muscle groups evenly.

When you do weight-bearing – or resistance – exercises your muscles take the strain. Repetitive motion tires and exhausts them, causing tiny tears in the muscle fibres. As your body repairs the damage, the fibres thicken and the muscles become stronger. However, this doesn't mean that you'll get bulky muscles by following the programme – quite the opposite, in fact. As fat gets replaced by lean muscle you'll begin to see a more defined shape as key areas tone up – your waist, upper arms and even your inner thighs will shrink. Big muscles only result from lifting big weights.

the importance of rest

Muscles need a day to rest after each toning session. This is essential because without recovery time the body can't repair muscle fibres. Continuous resistance exercise day after day can weaken muscles, affecting performance, and possibly causing injury. Bear in mind that on 'rest days', when you power walk rather than tone, your muscles are getting stronger. Your body doesn't atrophy just because you're not doing a resistance workout – you're getting stronger and fitter. Good-quality sleep will also help your body's ability to rest and regenerate (see pages 56–7).

the water factor

Water, the basis of our bloodstream, delivers necessary oxygen (in our red blood cells) and nutrients (in our plasma) to the body's vital organs, so keeping hydrated helps your muscles to work more efficiently as they get the liquid fuel they need. It's vital that you keep your body hydrated by drinking enough water – eight or nine glasses a day are recommended just to replace natural fluid loss. If you're exercising, you will need more – drink an extra glass or two for every half-hour that you exercise.

Never wait until you're thirsty before drinking – thirst is a sign that you are already dehydrated. Many people find it hard to drink water consistently and often lose track of how much they've drunk. To monitor your intake, fill a two-litre bottle with water each morning and drink from it throughout the day. If you're trying to lose weight as well as tone up, nutritionists recommend increasing water intake to cleanse your system of natural waste products, boost energy levels and improve your complexion.

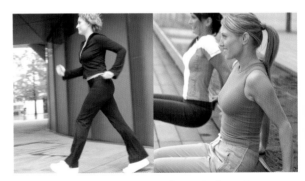

When you perform exercises such as walking, cycling, running and swimming, you use your muscles to accelerate.

When you do toning exercises your muscles are working by resisting an external weight or your own body weight.

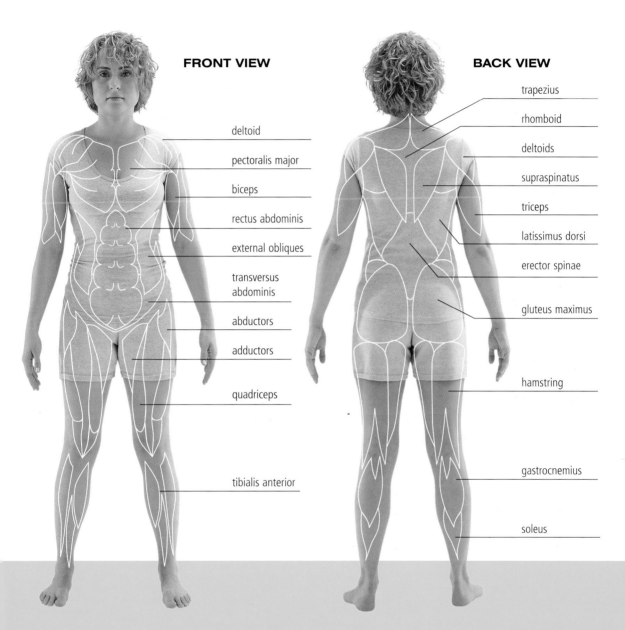

FRONT VIEW

deltoid

pectoralis major

biceps

rectus abdominis

external obliques

transversus abdominis

abductors

adductors

quadriceps

tibialis anterior

BACK VIEW

trapezius

rhomboid

deltoids

supraspinatus

triceps

latissimus dorsi

erector spinae

gluteus maximus

hamstring

gastrocnemius

soleus

the body's major muscle groups

The body contains hundreds of muscles – those shown here are
the major muscle groups, which are prime calorie burners.

better diet, better body
balancing the basics

The key to a great body and better health is balance. This may sound all too familiar, but a balanced diet, with enough fresh fruit, vegetables, carbohydrate and protein is critical for good health and weight management. Yet so often, when fat-fighting with fad diets it's all too easy to lose sight of the nutrition basics that really work. Here's how you can lose weight healthily – just by eating the right foods more often.

why diets don't work

Most fad or crash diets don't work – either you don't lose weight or if you do succeed, any significant weight loss can't be maintained for longer than a few weeks. This is because many diets involve deprivation, which conflicts with your body's primitive survival instincts. Your body retreats into fat-storing starvation mode. Calorie-burning, lean muscle tissue gets used for fuel, while unwanted fat stays put as your body conserves it in readiness for famine. In effect, you store up fat and cannibalise your own muscle as interim 'food'. Your metabolism slows down, and your blood-sugar level plummets, leaving you feeling lethargic, with low concentration levels.

Even if you've managed to lose some weight by dieting this way, when you start eating normally again your lowered metabolic rate is the reason why you usually gain weight so quickly – and all that deprivation feels pointless. It can be easy to become trapped in this type of fad-diet cycle, when you cannot maintain a healthy, steady weight without yo-yo dieting.

Eating regularly actually helps you to lose weight; some nutritionists recommend eating every three hours as a way to speed up metabolism. This is because eating smaller meals throughout the day, rather than building up to a grand dinner each night, drives your body into regular digestive action, burning off more calories. Eat regular, healthy meals and you'll have the edge, both metabolically and mentally.

keep it simple

I believe in keeping food simple. Eating balanced meals that include carbohydrates, protein-rich foods and plenty of fruits and vegetables speeds up weight loss and improves health. It works for me, and for my clients.

Try to eat five portions of fruits and vegetables a day – a total of 450g (1lb). This measure, recommended by the World Health Organisation and advocated in the UK in 1998 by the Department of Health, was introduced thanks to growing medical evidence that eating fruits and vegetables protects against some cancers, heart disease and other chronic conditions, such as type 2 diabetes, as well as helping to reduce the symptoms of asthma and diabetes. Potatoes, as well as yams, cassava and plantain, count as a starchy food and are best considered over and above your five a day. You can eat a combination of fresh, frozen, canned and dried fruits and vegetables.

To get even more vitamins and minerals, you could add in fruit juices or vegetable juices as one portion each day. A vegetable juicer is a great investment, enabling you to juice

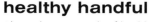

hard vegetables and fruits such as carrot, beetroot and apple in minutes. You'll also find it can be much cheaper to make your own juices than it is to buy ready-made. Here are some suggested juice combinations for an enlivening morning drink or afternoon pick-me-up:

• Carrot and a little fresh ginger root
• Apple with a little celery
• Cucumber and apple

Whenever you can, avoid foods with high levels of saturated fats and refined sugar. Unfortunately, these may include many of the foods you love, such as full-fat cheese on toast (which is high in saturated fat) or gooey carrot cake. Don't exclude these foods completely, but do restrict yourself to a half-portion and, whenever possible, use a delaying tactic if you are tempted to snack on them: drink some water, distract yourself for 15 minutes or so by making a telephone call, washing up, checking emails – anything that focuses your mind. If you're still craving a snack after this time, allow yourself something healthy (see pages 40–1).

eat slowly

Whatever you eat, always eat it slowly and savour every mouthful. The brain takes some time to register when you are full – around 20 minutes. Wait for your brain to catch up with your stomach, and you'll find that you eat a little less when dining out.

I often use this idea when I'm tempted to order a pudding. In many restaurants we're shown the dessert menu within 20 minutes of finishing the main course, during which time it can be easy to think that we're still hungry, and with encouragement could just make room for a little something extra. However, I tend to find that if I wait 20 minutes before thinking about dessert, I don't need or want sweet treats. Try it – it works!

healthy handful

Always keep a supply of healthy snacks close at hand.

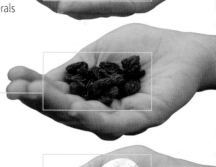

nuts have a high energy value thanks to their oil content

seeds contain many essential vitamins and minerals

raisins provide a great high-energy, low-fat snack

rice cakes are low in fat and handy for carrying with you

FIVE PORTIONS A DAY SUGGESTION

1 Breakfast Defrosted mixed berries with yogurt

2 Lunch Salad of your choice, containing a portion of mixed salad leaves and some beans

3 Dinner Carrot and coriander soup

4–5 Fresh steamed broccoli, cabbage or kale with frozen peas and protein of your choice

Snacks: banana, apple, dried apricots

eat breakfast, burn calories

If there's just one thing you can do to help control your weight, it's eating breakfast. When you don't eat early, there's a greater tendency to eat late, by which time you're more likely to be sedentary and burning fewer calories. Even a light breakfast, such as a banana or a handful of sunflower seeds stirred into a yogurt will rev up your blood sugar and protect you from mid-morning munchies.

Research shows that not only do people who don't eat breakfast eventually consume more calories throughout the course of the day than those who do, but also that the foods they eat are less likely to meet two-thirds of their body's other nutritional requirements. This may be because not eating first thing can lead to extreme hunger, which results in poor food choices, such as sweet muffins, fat-laden croissants, chocolate bars or a bacon sandwich instead of nutritious alternatives.

good breakfast choices These include:
• Poached, boiled or scrambled eggs on wholemeal or seeded toast – a great protein/carb-balanced meal that keeps you going all morning.

• Fruit smoothies – make one by blending fruits such as oranges, apples, bananas and berries with natural yogurt. As an alternative, or if you're vegan, opt for silken tofu instead of yogurt, which also gives you a protein hit and keeps you feeling fuller for longer.
• Oats, which are rich in heart-protective soluble fibre. Add a dessertspoonful of mixed pumpkin and sunflower seeds and serve with water or soya milk. You can also add berries to provide an extra daily portion of fruit (for convenience, buy frozen blueberries, blackberries, raspberries, strawberries and cranberries). Alternatively, make porridge with milk or water and stir the seeds and fruit into it once cooked.
• Organic muesli (choose one with low sugar and salt content) followed by fresh fruit.

plan ahead

It's vital to plan what you eat each day to ensure you get the right balance of nutrition you need. When you don't think ahead, your food standards can go downhill. For example, if you forget to take a healthy snack with you on a train journey at 6pm, by the time you arrive at your destination at 7pm you are so ravenous that you'll happily

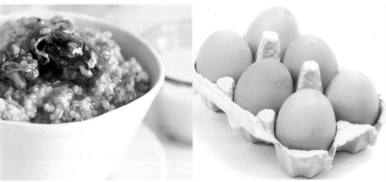

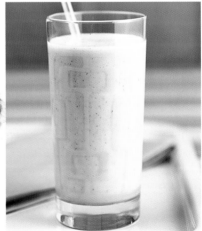

Breakfast is a must for boosting your metabolism first thing in the morning. Rather than make do with whatever you find in the fridge, plan your breakfasts in advance and enjoy a variety of foods as you kickstart your day.

feast on any food you can lay your hands on. With your blood-sugar levels descending by the minute, you might opt for a stodgy takeaway that has little nutritional value. And all because you didn't get the right food at 6pm.

Treat yourself well by having healthy snacks to hand at all times – keep supplies in your handbag and desk drawer so that wherever you go you won't be dependent on fast food that you wouldn't choose otherwise. Rice cakes, crumpets, fresh or dried fruit and home-made popcorn are low fat and will keep you going. Use them to fuel your workout, too (see page 41).

what to drink?

water benefits Drink eight or more glasses of water a day to keep your body hydrated. Symptoms of dehydration include headache, fatigue and irritability. If you are thirsty, it's a sign that you are already dehydrated and, just as with hunger, you body begins to fear deprivation and takes remedial action. Drinking plenty of water has many benefits:

• helps your body to eliminate toxins
• regulates temperature
• improves your skin condition
• helps you to exercise more efficiently.

what about coffee? Studies have shown that caffeine before exercise can have some mild performance benefits because it acts as a stimulant and improves fuel use. However, drinking lots of coffee can cause headaches, stomach upsets or anxiety in some people. It also has a diuretic effect, which can cause dehydration. I always advise my clients to drink water throughout the day and to choose diluted fresh juices and herbal teas rather than caffeine drinks such as coffee, stimulant drinks and colas. Having too much caffeine can also interfere with your sleep (see pages 56–7).

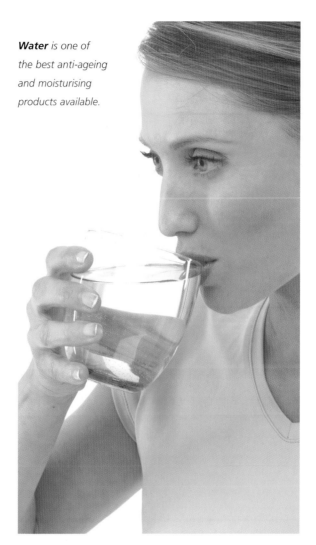

Water is one of the best anti-ageing and moisturising products available.

'Always eat breakfast to kickstart your metabolism in the morning. Cleanse your system by drinking a glass or two of cool water, or have warm water with lemon for a cosy start to a cold day.'

20 amazing benefits
of your workout

If you are struggling to get motivated and start exercising, the benefits listed below will encourage you to get moving. And your body will quickly reward you as lethargy is replaced by increasing energy levels and an overall improved sense of wellbeing.

20 benefits

1 Helps you to lose weight

2 Improves your co-ordination

3 Helps you to stand taller

4 Improves your flexibility

5 Helps you to sleep better and longer

6 Increases your metabolic rate and therefore your energy levels

7 Increases your lung capacity

8 Helps to maintain healthy muscles, bones and joints

9 Firms and tones your body all over

10 Improves your mood

11 Increases your confidence levels

12 Keeps you looking younger for longer

13 Keeps your appetite under control

14 Helps you to feel more in control of your life

15 Makes your hair, skin and nails gleam

16 Improves your sports performance

17 Reduces your stress levels

18 Helps to decrease the frequency and severity of hot flushes

19 Helps to prevent osteoporosis

20 Improves your attitude to everything else in your life!

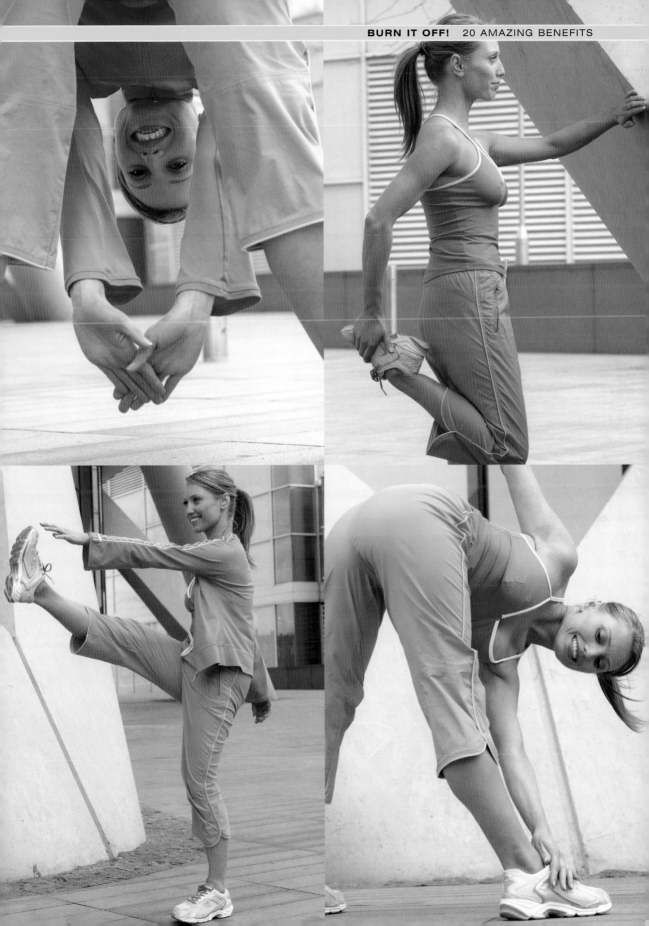

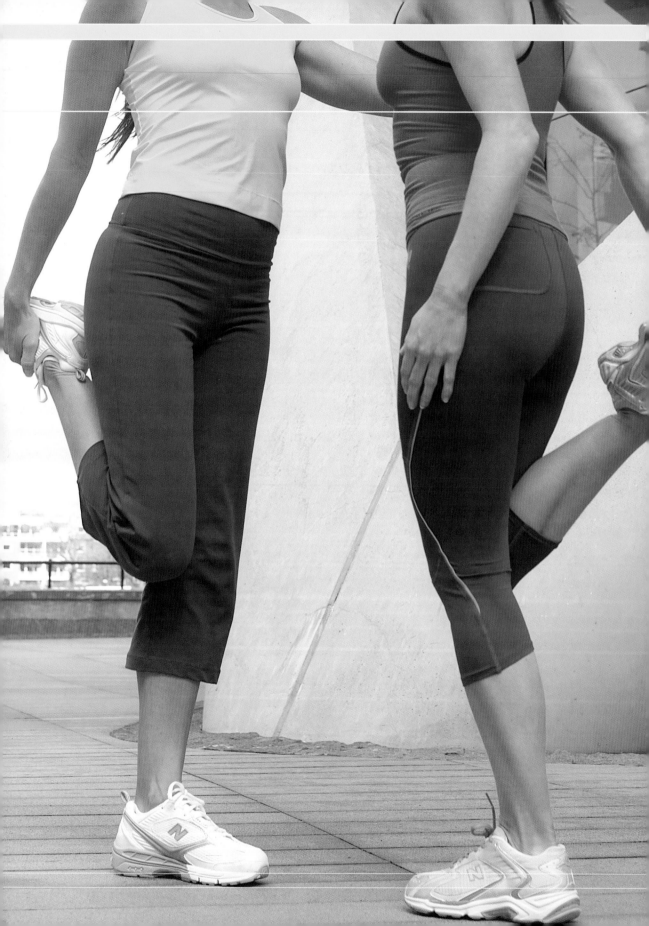

get into the programme

building up to exercise

Now that you have decided to get into the No-Gym Workout, you need to get ready on a practical level before you can start. First, gather together any equipment you might need for exercising, whether at home, outdoors or at work, paying special attention to staying safe while exercising. Next, you need to think about when is the best time to exercise, on a day-to-day basis as well as making the most of your naturally energetic periods. And finally, determine your power walking programme. Now you are ready to get started.

how the no-gym workout works
where to begin

Start by deciding how you can fit the No-Gym Workout into your lifestyle. Then you can learn how best to measure your progress, prepare for power walking and get wise on safety, stretching and when to work out. Establish what equipment you'll need for your home gym – the minimum investment is a good pair of trainers, but you can also buy resistance bands, workout clothes and even a Swiss ball (see page 30).

the power of three

The No-Gym Workout focuses on doing three different exercises per week – each of which you do three times during that week – alternating daily with power walks. The exercises are simple, but precise, and they are designed to target the major muscle groups. They fall into three categories – upper body, middle body and lower body. You do one exercise from each category for week one,

then a different set from each category for week two, and so on, until by the end of week six you have toned all the major muscles in your body. The categories are colour-coded for ease of reference (see below).

measuring up Before you begin the programme, take your measurements. Unless you really can't be parted from your scales, don't weigh yourself – measurements

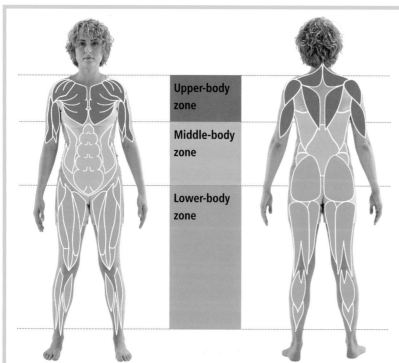

Upper-body zone

Middle-body zone

Lower-body zone

THE BODY ZONES

The upper-body exercises tone the shoulders and arms and lift and firm the bust – rescue for flabby upper arms and sinking cleavage.

The middle-body exercises tone the stomach, waist and buttocks – great for improving core stability, protecting your back, defining your waist and firming a wobbly tummy and bottom.

The lower-body exercises tone the legs and ankles – giving you great legs and more strength in your lower body.

reflect your shape, whereas weight can be misleading because you'll be gaining muscle in strategic areas and as muscle weighs more than fat, you may find that even though you're in better shape your weight may increase. What really matters to most of my clients is being able to look good and feel confident in the clothes they choose to wear, whether it's an outfit for a special occasion or everyday wear. Choose an item of clothing you're yearning to get back into – a pair of jeans is a popular choice – and use this as a yardstick of your progress.

• Take your bust, waist and hip measurements once a week and try on your chosen clothing item once a week, too.

• Pay special attention to your vital statistics at week three, as this is when you'll begin to see a real change.

• Add your measurements to the checklist at the end of each week's exercises (see pages 57, 69, 81, 93, 105, 117).

planning your week People often give up exercising because they feel demotivated by repeating the same workout programme. By varying your routine every week (see below) you'll never grow bored. You can also mix

and match the exercises – just choose one upper-, middle- and lower-body exercise from any week. And when the six weeks are up, continue to enjoy a variety of exercises by devising your own sequence (see pages 134–5).

boosting the burn Once you find you can do 20 repetitions of an exercise with relative ease, you are ready to increase the intensity, thus burning more calories. Each exercise in the programme has a boost the burn alternative, describing how to take the exercise to the next level. The figures given for the number of calories burned for each exercise refer only to the basic exercise.

reap the rewards What is wonderfully simple and practical about this workout is that you don't need lots of specialist equipment to do it – you can change your body shape and reclaim your vitality by getting back to basics. Neither do you need to spend hours of your precious time working out. Just follow these clever, precise moves for six weeks, enjoy regular power walks (see page 34–7) and eat a healthy, balanced diet to achieve results.

	Week 1	Week 2
Monday	Tone	Walk
Tuesday	Walk	Tone
Wednesday	Tone	Walk
Thursday	Walk	Tone
Friday	Tone	Walk
Saturday	Walk	Tone
Sunday	Rest	Rest

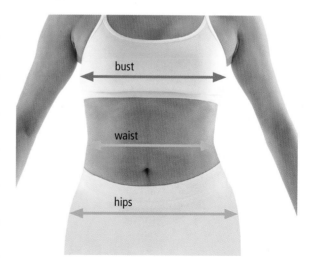

Measure your bust, waist and hips once a week to chart your progress – you will quickly notice how your shape is changing.

useful equipment
the no-gym wish list

Plan for starting your workout by gathering the clothes and the tools you need to help you feel motivated and look good. Getting organised in advance helps to reconfirm your commitment to yourself and to the programme, and increases the chances that you will remain focused for the full six weeks and beyond. All the following pieces of equipment are useful, although the only essential items are a good pair of trainers and a mat.

exercise aids

pedometer A pedometer calculates steps and distance (see pages 34–7). Sophisticated models calculate calories burned using weight, distance and pulse rate, but a simple model is good enough for the No-Gym Workout.

resistance bands Resistance bands are one of the best fitness products around. Used in healthcare – physiotherapists use them to redress injury – they have become the totem of the pilates class as well as strength training. Featured in some of the higher-intensity exercises in this book, these latex bands are lightweight and highly effective – they work your muscles four times harder by increasing resistance created by your body weight.

Resistance bands come in different colours to denote how much resistance they give. Pink usually has least resistance and generally has the right intensity for women. Other colours depend on the manufacturers, who have different colour-coding systems, but often green, yellow and purple bands are increasingly resistant, topped by a super-strong black band suitable only for the extremely athletic.

hand weights You can buy hand weights for your workouts and power walking (see pages 34–5). If you're a beginner, start with 500ml water bottles rather than buying 1kg or 1.5kg weights that you'll soon grow out of. Begin by filling the water bottles half-full and work towards full bottles as you grow stronger. Once you have reasonably

good upper-body fitness, buy some 2kg weights. Stick with these, otherwise you'll gain bulk on your upper arms rather than lean definition.

swiss ball The Swiss ball is becoming so familiar in homes that it is almost part of the furniture – but do make sure that you remember to use it. Working with a Swiss ball (also known as a stability ball) improves strength and core stability because when you sit on it or perform other exercises your body has to engage extra muscles, including the abdominals, to hold you in place. You can even give yourself a mini-workout by sitting on your ball rather than the sofa while you watch television.

sports bra Wear a sports bra when you power walk. The level of intensity you'll be walking at will be higher than the level you use for regular walking, so you need to protect breast tissue from stretching, which over time can cause the bust to sag. If you can, get measured for a sports bra because wearing the wrong size can mean you won't get the right support for your breasts.

trainers Choose trainers that fit well when wearing one pair of trainer socks. Cushioning in the heel is a must, because when you power walk each step impacts through the heel. Ankles must have good padding, too – they are delicate and it's easy to damage them if your trainers don't give adequate protection. Ignore brands, and go for comfort and cushioned support first and foremost.

your home gym

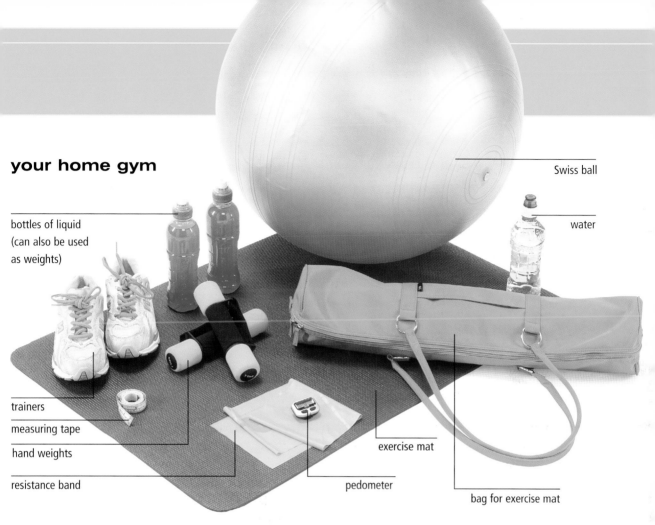

Swiss ball

bottles of liquid
(can also be used
as weights)

water

trainers

measuring tape

hand weights

resistance band

pedometer

exercise mat

bag for exercise mat

clothes While toning at home, you might enjoy not having to dress for the gym, so wear whatever you feel comfortable in, as long as it allows a full range of movement. As you progress, you may choose to wear fitted exercise tops and leggings to appreciate your body as you tone up. When you power walk, good quality workout gear will also keep you ventilated while keeping your muscles warm. Wearing layers will help you to stay cool during your walk. If you power walk after dark (see page 43) always wear a reflective vest.

mirror A mirror helps you to see that you're doing each exercise correctly, and in particular helps to check the position of your pelvis, back and shoulders. Using two facing mirrors allows you to see yourself easily from two angles, rather than straining your neck trying. Alternatively, ask a friend to be your mirror by watching your exercises

and advising you of any necessary adjustment. Always be guided by what feels comfortable.

exercise mat Exercise mats are cushioned to protect your joints and other bones from hard flooring, and some are lightly ribbed to prevent slippage. Lay down a clean towel if you don't have a mat. Placing your mat or towel and setting up your mirrors, if you have them, can become part of your ritual before you begin exercising. Rituals help you to change mode mentally and physically, preparing you for your workout.

music Each week, choose mood-lifting music to accompany your toning exercises. Music is a great motivator, which is why gyms play constant, high-energy music. Create your home-gym atmosphere by playing any CDs that inspire you and make you feel energised.

warming up, cooling down
preparations for exercise

Warming up before and cooling down after you tone or power walk is the best possible preparation for exercise. This is because stretching your muscles before and after intense activity not only helps you achieve a full range of motion, it also prevents that aching-all-over feeling the next day – and, vitally, protects your body from injury.

When muscles are cold or resting, they contract; when they are warm and active, they expand. So the purpose of a warm-up sequence is to expand the muscles using gentle movement, ready for intensive action. Always warm up before you stretch, even if you just march on the spot for two minutes. You need to cool down after exercise, too, to help the muscles gradually contract back into rest mode.

calf muscles Step forward about 30cm (1ft) or so, bending your knee. Lean forward from your hips, keeping your back straight and your navel pulled in towards your spine. Keep your heels down and your elbows back, with your hands resting on your hips or leaning against a tree. Hold for a count of five, and then repeat on the other leg.

hamstrings Bend one knee and extend the other leg in front of you, with your foot flexed and heel to the floor. Rest both palms on the supporting thigh – not on the thigh of your extended leg, as this can push your knees into the 'locked out' position. Keep your abdominal muscles pulled in tight. Now stick out your tailbone to enhance the stretch through the hamstring muscle of the extended leg. Hold for a count of five, then change legs.

quadriceps Stand with your feet hip-width apart. Pull in your abdominal muscles to help you to balance as you catch hold of one ankle and pull gently to stretch the quadricep muscles on the front of the thigh. Hold for five seconds and release. Repeat on the opposite leg.

upper arms and shoulders Stand with your feet hip-width apart. Your spine should be neutral – straight and relaxed. Clasp your hands in front of you at chest level, so your arms form an arc as you allow a gentle pull across the top of your back, stretching the trapezius muscles. Keep your navel pulled in towards your spine, and your knees soft.

chest Stand with your feet hip-width apart with neutral spine and soft knees. Pull in your abdominal muscles. Clasp your hands behind your back and raise them until you feel the stretch across your chest and down your arms. Don't let your back arch – keep it supported by pulling your navel towards your spine. Look straight ahead, and keep your shoulders down. Hold for five seconds.

triceps Stand with your feet hip-width apart, knees slightly bent. Raise one of your arms and place your hand over your back. Try to reach as far down the midline of your spine as possible. Increase the stretch by gently pulling your elbow with your other hand.

THE BENEFITS OF STRETCHING

- Improves flexibility

- Prevents injury – failure to warm up is the biggest single cause of sports injury

- Prepares you mentally for a workout by giving you time to shift from work or domestic mindset to exercise mode

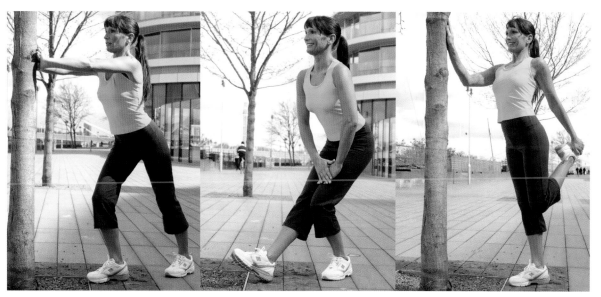

Calf muscle stretch Keep your back straight and your navel pulled in towards your spine as you stretch.

Hamstring stretch Rest both palms on the supporting thigh and feel the stretch all the way down the back of the other thigh.

Quadricep stretch Hold one ankle and pull gently. You will feel the stretch down the front of your thigh.

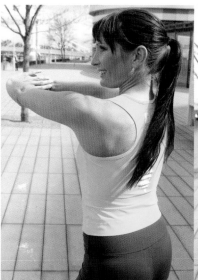

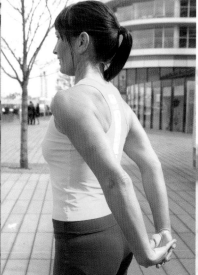

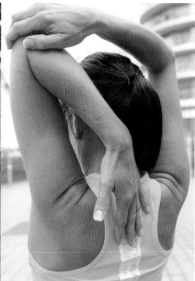

Upper arms, shoulders and top of back stretch Keep your spine neutral and clasp your hands in front of you at chest level.

Chest stretch Clasp your hands together behind your back and raise them until you feel the stretch.

Triceps stretch Extend and bend your arm so you touch the top of your back. Gently pull the elbow with your other hand.

power walking
work it off

Power walking helps to melt away unwanted fat as it raises your metabolic rate, boosting your body's calorie-burning potential. Start by power walking for 20 minutes at a time, three times a week. And remember, the more you walk, the more energy you'll have. All you need to do is plan your route then get started – and believe me, once you get going, you'll love the stimulus to your mind and body.

how to power walk

When you power walk, you need to walk at a speed that leaves you slightly out of breath – on the Borg scale (see page 43) aim for level 5, working somewhat hard, and maintain this throughout the walk. Walk through the full length of your feet, from the heel to the toe, and use your arms. Don't carry anything – use a waist purse, tiny back pack or pockets for essentials such as your keys, mobile phone and water (see the safety notes on pages 42–3). Your arms need to be able to move freely, and to carry small hand weights, if you prefer.

• Hold your abdominal muscles in as you walk – ideally, engage them so they feel pulled about one-third of the way towards the spine. To gauge this level, relax your stomach muscles completely, and practise holding them in in three stages. At stage one all your muscles are engaged but not tight, at stage two you're about halfway, and at stage three you're pulling your tummy in as far as you can. Aim to walk at stage one, so your stomach muscles feel firm but allow you to breathe deeply. As you power walk, you'll be giving your abs a mini-workout, too.

• Keep your shoulders back and down. Don't tense up as you walk. This can happen when you have that feeling that you need to get the walk 'over with'. When you're in this kind of resistance mode, doing something because you feel you have to rather than because you want to, it shows up in your body language – your fists clench and your muscles

tense, particularly in your neck and back. If you feel like this when you first power walk, just focus on your breathing to release stress (see below). Always walk in safety (see pages 42–3). If you don't feel comfortable in your environment, you won't enjoy power walking.

Many people enjoy power walking because it is revitalising and refreshing, as well as providing an opportunity to destress both mind and body.

breathing You'll get more benefits from your walks by breathing deeply (see pages 104–5). If you are holding in your abdominal muscles too much you may tense up and chest-breathe (using only your upper lungs). Breathe in deeply through your nose and out through your mouth, taking the air down into your lower lungs. This oxygenates your blood, giving you energy, and promotes relaxation.

LUCY'S TIP

Whatever your pedometer reading (see page 36), motivate yourself by rounding it up to the nearest 100 steps. Get a competition going at home – encourage others you live with to aim for a weekly step goal and keep a chart on the fridge recording everyone's achievements.

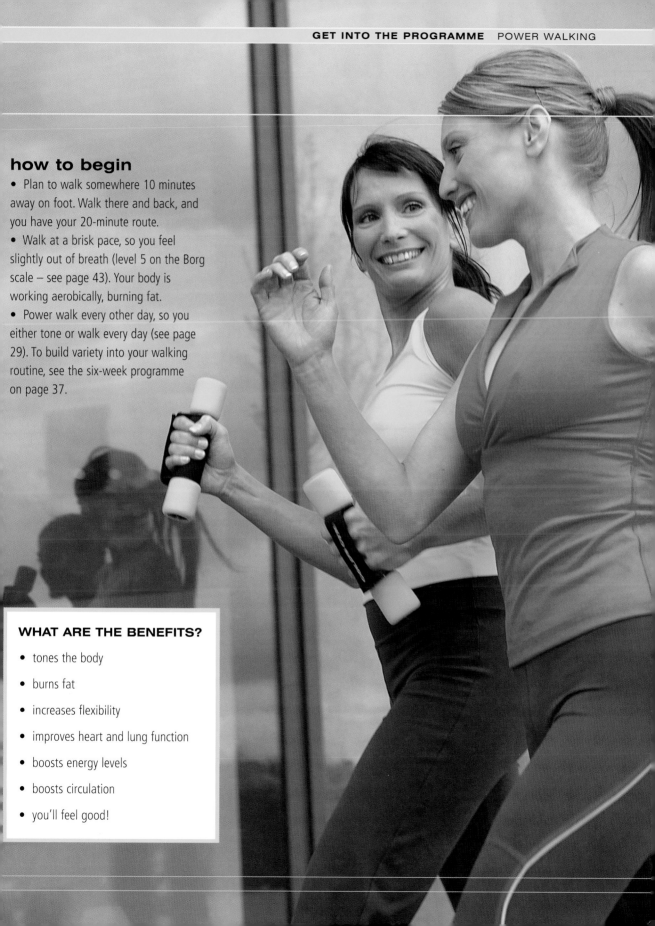

how to begin

- Plan to walk somewhere 10 minutes away on foot. Walk there and back, and you have your 20-minute route.
- Walk at a brisk pace, so you feel slightly out of breath (level 5 on the Borg scale – see page 43). Your body is working aerobically, burning fat.
- Power walk every other day, so you either tone or walk every day (see page 29). To build variety into your walking routine, see the six-week programme on page 37.

WHAT ARE THE BENEFITS?

- tones the body
- burns fat
- increases flexibility
- improves heart and lung function
- boosts energy levels
- boosts circulation
- you'll feel good!

getting the best results
maximising benefits

Motivation, as ever, is key. An early power walk is metabolically beneficial, and also good psychology: start the day as you mean to go on, putting health and fitness first. If you can, plan to power walk in the morning or at lunchtime, as the earlier in the day you exercise, the sooner you raise your metabolic rate. If the only time you can power walk is after 5pm, fuel up with a healthy snack before you go (see pages 40–1).

motivational monitoring

A pedometer is a great motivational tool and a reliable way to monitor every step you take. This device contains a ball bearing that moves backwards and forwards as you walk, giving a step count. It clips on to your waistband above the hip, from which point it can monitor motion. Wear your pedometer all day, every day – your total steps per day (see below) can include every step you take, from walking to the bathroom to running a mile.

how many steps? Most active adults take a minimum of 5000–6000 steps a day. To lose weight and really improve fitness, aim for 10,000 or more, and a grand weekly total of 80,000 steps. Ten thousand steps equals about 8km (5 miles), so in a week you could cover 65km (40 miles) on foot. Think creatively about how to increase your activity level, such as walking instead of driving for short shopping trips or walking halfway to work. Keep a note of your steps per week and add them to the checklists that appear at the end of every week's exercises (see pages 57, 69, 81, 93, 105, 117).

burn it off with hand weights

Use hand weights and you'll burn up to 40 per cent more calories. Carrying them as you walk makes your body work harder, creating more resistance as your body pushes against the weight to propel you forward. Hand weights are also a great way to get an upper-body workout as you walk, toning the triceps, biceps, chest and shoulders.

Always use light hand weights for power walks, no matter how you feel physically before you begin. Just like shopping bags, what feels light enough for the first five or 10 minutes can transform quickly into a lead weight after 20. And you'll have no choice but to keep carrying the weight until you reach your car or your doorstep, potentially damaging your muscles. I find the best way to begin with weights is to use water bottles (500ml), because if you overestimate what you can carry you can always drink the water or pour some away to lighten the load. Later, you can progress to 2kg weights (see page 30) but this is the absolute maximum, unless you want to use heavier weights to build muscle bulk, which is beyond the remit of this book.

To use hand weights while walking, hold each weight firmly lengthways with your palms facing in. As you raise each weight during your natural walking action, don't allow the weight to go any further than chest height, at which point the upper arm muscles will be fully contracted so the action (and benefit of the exercise) is complete.

different terrains

Once you become an accomplished power walker, increase the intensity of your walks by diverting away from the roads and pavements – which are smoother and therefore easier to walk on – and try some different terrains. Power walking across country works the leg muscles harder, and hills are great for toning the bottom and legs, as well as improving fitness and stamina.

POWER WALKING PROGRAMME

Here's how to vary and extend your power walks over the six-week training period. To begin, all you have to do is walk out of your front door, keep going for 10 minutes, then walk back. You'll burn off an average of approximately 124 calories each time you power walk. Progress to interval training, using hand weights as well as adding an extra 10 minutes to your route, and you'll be burning approximately 191 calories.

week 1: Just starting
Aim for three power walks of 20 minutes each, walking at a fast pace so it feels somewhat hard (level 5 on the Borg scale – see page 43).

week 2: Set the pace
Plan a one-mile route – measure the distance by car. Walk it, noting the time its takes you. For the next two or three power walks repeat the route, trying to take minutes off the clock.

week 3: Interval train
Walk for three minutes at level 5 (somewhat hard) so you feel slightly out of breath, then walk

for one minute as fast as you can, then go back to walking at level 5 for three minutes. Do this for the whole 20-minute walk. Interval training adds variation and helps to keep your focus, while also boosting the burn and adding to the challenge of the exercise.

week 4: Go to thirty
You're over halfway through the programme, so you should be feeling a real difference by now. Aim for a 30-minute power walk, three times a week, at level 5.

week 5: Use hand weights
Because you'll be burning 40 per cent more calories using hand weights (see facing page), reduce the time of your power walks from 30 to 25 minutes.

week 6: Hill challenge
This week, add in hills – find a new route with hills and walk for 25 minutes at level 5 with hand weights. By now, you should be feeling super fit. See how far you've come by going back to the one-mile route from Week 2 and time how fast you walk it now compared to your Week 2 record.

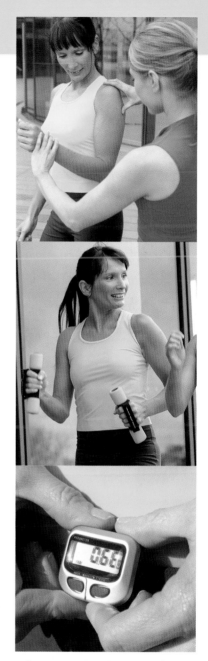

When you're power walking, your arms should be bent, forming an L-shape (top). **Using hand weights** *burns more calories and tones the backs of your arms (middle).* **Wear your pedometer** *all day and aim for at least 10,000 steps per day (above).*

tuning into your monthly cycle
get into the rhythm

Over the course of an average 28-day menstrual cycle, hormonal changes impact on our energy levels. Intuitively, we respond to these subtle or marked energetic changes that occur throughout our cycle. However, being more aware of your energy highs and lows can help you to work with your body, maximising energy surges and managing more easily the down-times when energy is in short supply.

days 1–5: menstruation

Should you work out during your period? Old wives' tales tell us not to do all sorts of things, such as wash our hair, never mind venturing out for a power walk. Yet I find many of my clients benefit from doing some exercise at this time, and exercises you might shy away from are actually those that can help ease menstrual discomfort the most. Any sit-up exercise, which focuses on toning the abdominals, can for some women ease period pain. If you can manage this, fine, but if you feel too uncomfortable, opt for a brisk power walk to boost your circulation and lift your mood.

days 6–14: oestrogen rising

Between days 6 and 13, oestrogen levels rise, culminating in ovulation on around day 14 of the cycle, when a mature egg is released from the ovaries. Oestrogen is also the hormone responsible for sex drive. Consequently, many women feel more vital, creative and outgoing at this time, and can also experience heightened sexual confidence. During this rising phase, you'll generally have more energy, but don't be tempted to take on more work and social activity as these can, in turn, interfere with your toning time and power walks. You may need a little more willpower

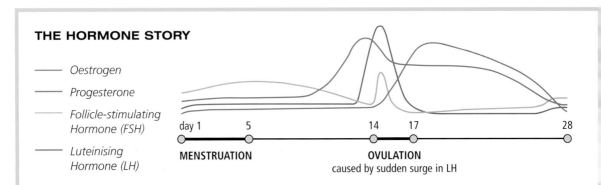

THE HORMONE STORY

—— *Oestrogen*

—— *Progesterone*

—— *Follicle-stimulating Hormone (FSH)*

—— *Luteinising Hormone (LH)*

day 1   5   14   17   28

MENSTRUATION

OVULATION
caused by sudden surge in LH

Four hormones interact during the menstural cycle: follicle-stimulating hormone (FSH), luteinising hormone (LH), oestrogen and progesterone. After your period has finished, FSH causes a mature egg to develop. The egg produces oestrogen and oestrogen levels rise during the first half of the cycle, peaking just before LH prompts ovulation, when the egg is released – usually around day 14. During the second half of the cycle progesterone is secreted, and the womb lining thickens in readiness to receive and nurture a fertilized egg. If fertilization doesn't occur, the thickened womb lining is lost each month during menstruation.

just now, so stick with your commitment to find time to exercise rather than succumbing to other distractions. You'll feel the benefit.

If you're weighing rather than measuring yourself during this programme (see page 29 for why measuring is preferable), mid-cycle is a good time to get on the scales. Some women suffer from water retention before their period, so weighing yourself in the week or few days leading up to menstruation can give an inaccurate reading.

days 15–26: fat melting, fat craving

My clients tell me that during this phase of their cycle exercising often feels easier and studies have shown that 30 per cent more fat is burnt. Just to make things a little more difficult, however, the increase of progesterone at this time can lead to increased food cravings, particularly close to the start of your period, so it can be harder to control your appetite for fatty, sugary chocolate, the pre-menstrual favourite. Your increased desire for chocolate may be due to lower magnesium levels at this point in your cycle. Try eating magnesium-rich broccoli and nuts instead.

days 27–28: energy surplus There also

appears to be much anecdotal evidence that women experience an energy rush a day or two before their period. This may manifest as the urge to do housework, perhaps because this feels like a natural time for cleansing and letting go, mirroring the process of menstruation. I believe that you can really improve your motivation by exercising when you feel that energy-burst – do housework by all means, but save a little energy for your toning exercises and power walking. When you begin your workout with an energy surfeit, you'll find you enjoy an even bigger adrenaline buzz, and the memory of this will help to get you through those lower points in your cycle when you are suffering from diminished motivation.

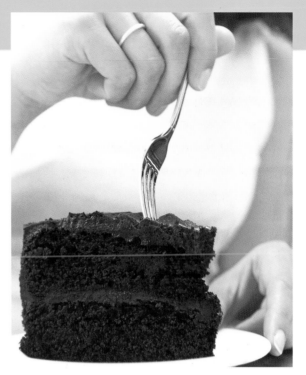

Sugar cravings needn't get the better of you – place your hands on this cake and with a little imagination it will magically absorb into your mouth, without a calorie in sight.

the wisdom of your cycle

The average 28-day menstrual cycle is often linked with the 28-day cycle of the moon, which is believed to influence the tides of the oceans and the fluids of our bodies. Some evidence suggests that many women's cycles synchronise with the moon phases, ovulating when the moon is full and menstruating during the waning moon and new moon.

Women's health expert Dr Christiane Northrup in her book *Women's Bodies, Women's Wisdom*, explains how the waxing moon (when the moon is growing to full size) is a time of expansion and creativity, and more physical energy, culminating in ovulation. The waning moon – when the moon is decreasing to its 'C' shape – can be a time of reflection during which, according to Dr Northrup, 'women are most in tune with their inner knowing and with what isn't working in their lives'. During the waning moon, women may also dream more vividly.

workout foods
healthy snacks

To get the best results from exercising and to make sure you have enough energy to enjoy working out and power walking, you need the right nutrition. Along with a healthy, balanced diet (see pages 20–3), plenty of sleep (see pages 56–7) and keeping hydrated, you also need to eat carbohydrates and proteins at the right times.

fuel your workout

Your body needs complex carbohydrates before you work out or power walk, and a mix of protein and carbs afterwards. This is because the body converts carbohydrates to glucose (blood sugar), which fuels your muscles and gives you the energy you need to exercise. However, don't eat a heavy meal before you exercise, and try to leave at least two hours between a main meal and a workout to give your body time to begin digestion. You can eat a light snack 30 minutes to an hour before beginning a workout. Complex carbohydrates include the following foods: wholegrain bread, porridge oats and cereals, pasta, couscous, rice (particularly brown rice), beans and pulses.

After your workout, eat some protein with carbohydrate. Protein builds and replenishes muscle, bones, skin and other body tissue, which is important when you've worked your muscles hard. Protein foods include meat (choose lean cuts), poultry, eggs, beans, fish and soya products, such as tofu, as well as dairy foods such as lower-fat milks, yogurts and cheeses. Remember also to aim to drink at least eight glasses of water a day (see page 23).

healthy snacking

It's important to choose the right snacks to keep your blood sugar even throughout the day, particularly when you're following an exercise programme. When your blood sugar dips, you are less likely to feel like doing your workout or power walk. However, if you keep your energy levels stable this gives you the energy you need to motivate yourself.

how to beat the comfort nibble

While it's a good idea to have a healthy snack before your workout, it can be easy to fuel up on snacks high in fat and/or sugar, believing that you'll work it off – or reward yourself with comfort treats post-workout. Although you do expend more calories while exercising, comfort eating in this way will ultimately sabotage your efforts. This doesn't mean you have to forego every treat, but it's important to be aware of just what you're eating – and if you need to eat it at all.

Before you put anything in your mouth, ask yourself how hungry you really are. Take the hunger test, scoring your level of hunger as follows:

1. Not hungry
2. Beginning to think about food – feeling bored
3. Would eat if someone offered you food
4. A little hungry – will check what's in the fridge/cupboard
5. Need a snack – concentration starting to suffer
6. Hungry
7. Very hungry
8. Starving

Eat if you genuinely feel you're at level 5 or above. Eating when you're at level 1, 2, 3 and 4, is officially comfort eating. To avoid this, create a time lapse between your hand and your mouth. Whenever you're not sure if you're truly hungry, drink a glass of water, go back to what you were doing for 15 minutes and reconsider. Often when you distract yourself your focus moves away from food and you realise you're not hungry after all.

SUPER SNACK RECIPES

pulse-starter
- One-third of a can of cannellini, haricot or butter beans
- 1 teaspoon olive oil
- Bread or bagel
- Tahini (optional)

Drain then mash the cold beans with the olive oil, and add the tahini (sesame seed paste). Tahini improves the quality of the protein in this snack by mixing the amino acids of the cannellini beans and sesame seeds. Season with a little pepper and spread on lightly toasted or fresh bread or bagel.

This snack is a great low-fat workout fuel, with a balanced carb and protein content.

popcorn
- 3 dessertspoons of maize
- 1 dessertspoon of olive oil

Add the oil to a hot pan, then add the maize and put on the pan lid. Leave for a minute or so, then shake the pan, keeping the lid in place, as the maize begins to pop. Allow to cool. Add salt or a little demerara sugar to make it savoury or sweet. For vanilla popcorn, add a vanilla pod after cooking.

The ultimate low-fat snacking food, popcorn is perfect after 9pm when you want something to munch that won't break your healthy eating plan.

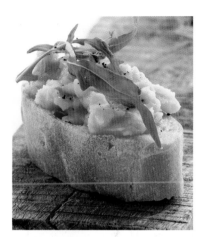

no-fat banana 'ice cream'
- One banana, medium soft

Peel the banana and place it in the freezer compartment until frozen. Mash the frozen banana and eat, or serve with a little fresh fruit, such as strawberries or raspberries.

I recommend banana ice cream to my clients because it really does rescue you from late-night doughnut fantasies.

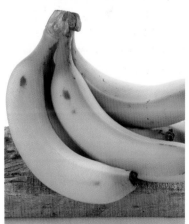

more pre-workout snacks
- half a bagel or rice cakes with hummous • crumpet, malt loaf, scones, teacake • oat or rice cakes, or cereal bars • breakfast cereal with semi-skimmed milk • fruit yogurt • toast or sandwich with peanut butter • a handful of sunflower seeds • a handful of nuts, raisins, apricots or dates • glass of skimmed milk or non-dairy alternative such as soya or rice milk • home-made vegetable soup • fruit smoothies made with low-fat natural yogurt or tofu (see page 22)

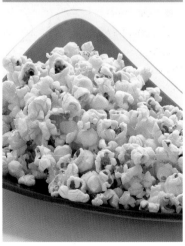

safe moves
keeping safety in mind

Safety should always be your first priority when exercising. When you feel safe and comfortable in your environment, indoors or outdoors, you relax and are able to enjoy your workout. Exercising with safety in mind, from knowing how to protect your back to how far to push yourself, allows you to tune into your body so you know how to get the most out of it, as well as being aware of your limitations.

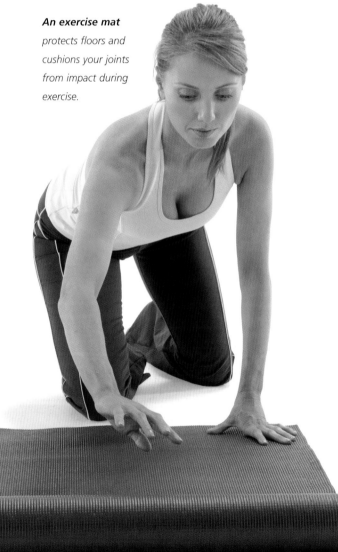

An exercise mat protects floors and cushions your joints from impact during exercise.

a safe environment

Create an exercise area that gives you plenty of room to move around in, and in which you won't bump into furniture or other potentially injurious items. While you won't be jogging around your home, you still need adequate space to extend your limbs – around 30cm (12in) or so beyond your outstretched toes and fingertips.

Use an exercise mat (see page 31) to support your joints – the cushioning a mat provides is preferable to a soft rug or carpet. A mat is essential if you have hard floors as the ribbed underside of the mat is designed to prevent slippage.

safety when power walking Here are a few important safety guidelines you should adhere to:
- Don't use an iPod – stay alert to your environment.
- Carry water with you.
- Wear a reflective vest if you're walking in the dark.
- Stick to main routes.
- Carry a mobile phone.
- Carry a whistle.
- Power walk with a friend – it's safer and more fun.

protect your back

Pull in your abdominal muscles during every exercise – imagine that you're pulling your navel tight to your spine. Keeping your stomach muscles tight improves core stability (the muscle tone in your abdomen and middle body), which protects your back from injury. Taut stomach muscles also improve your posture, helping you to stand taller as your back and upper body is fully supported.

breathe easy

It may sound obvious, but breathing correctly during exercise empowers your muscles by feeding them oxygen through the blood. It can be easy to forget to breathe evenly or deeply when you're concentrating on your posture, but using your breath energises your whole body and helps you to work harder (see pages 104–5).

In the programme, exercises that involve continuous motion such as the leg rotation (see page 100–1) require you to breathe evenly throughout. Others with an in-out, push-pull action require you to breathe at specific stages of the exercise. The general rule is to breathe out on the 'effort', and to breathe in on the return to the starting position.

find your level: the Borg scale

When you work out at the gym, you test your fitness by setting the machine to varying levels of difficulty. When you're at home, there's still an effective way to gauge

how far to push yourself when doing repetitions – it's less technical, but gets you more familiar with your personal abilities in a way in which no machine can. The scale is known as the Borg scale, and it is designed to measure your perceived rate of exertion:

1   Not exhausted at all
2   Extremely light effort required
3   Very light effort required
4   Moderately hard
5   Somewhat hard
6   Hard
7   Very hard
8   Extremely hard
9   Close to exhaustion
10 Total exhaustion

Level 5 is a good toning and fat-burning zone, so aim for this during your workout, although you will, of course, benefit from working out at level 4. Whenever you're exercising, ask yourself what level you're working at – be honest – and adjust your effort as you go to achieve a consistent 5 whenever you can.

WORKOUT DOS AND DON'TS

- Do always warm up before exercise.
- Do drink at least one glass of water before you begin.
- Do use a mat.
- Do pull in your abs to protect your back.
- Do breathe!
- Do wear a reflective vest when exercising outdoors.
- Don't exercise on a full stomach.
- Don't exercise if you're injured or feel unwell.
- Don't exercise if anything hurts.

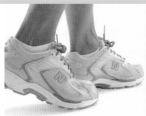
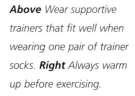
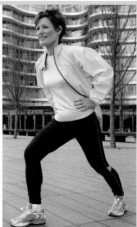

Above Wear supportive trainers that fit well when wearing one pair of trainer socks. **Right** Always warm up before exercising.

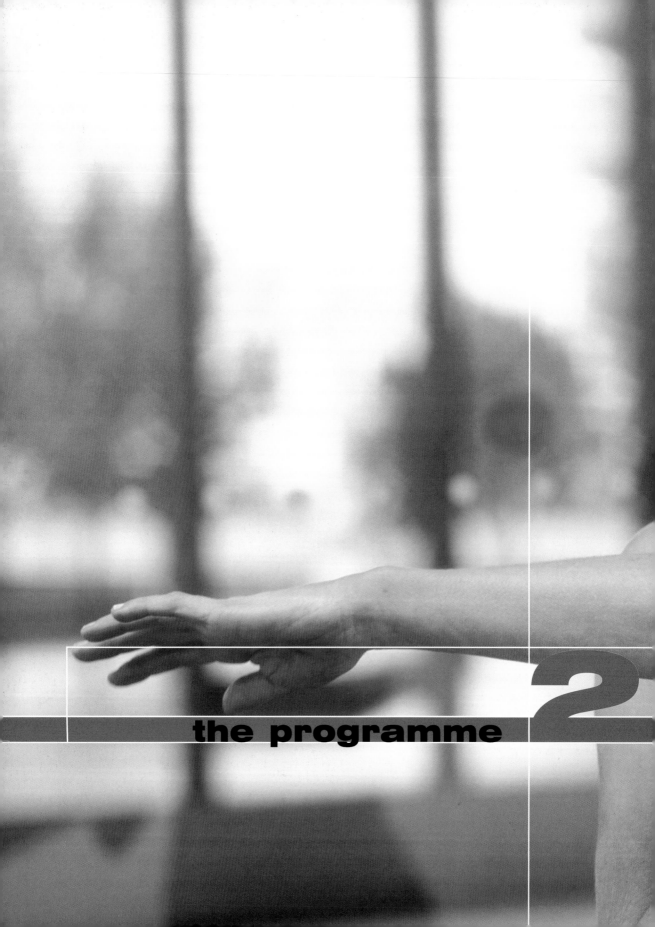

the programme 2

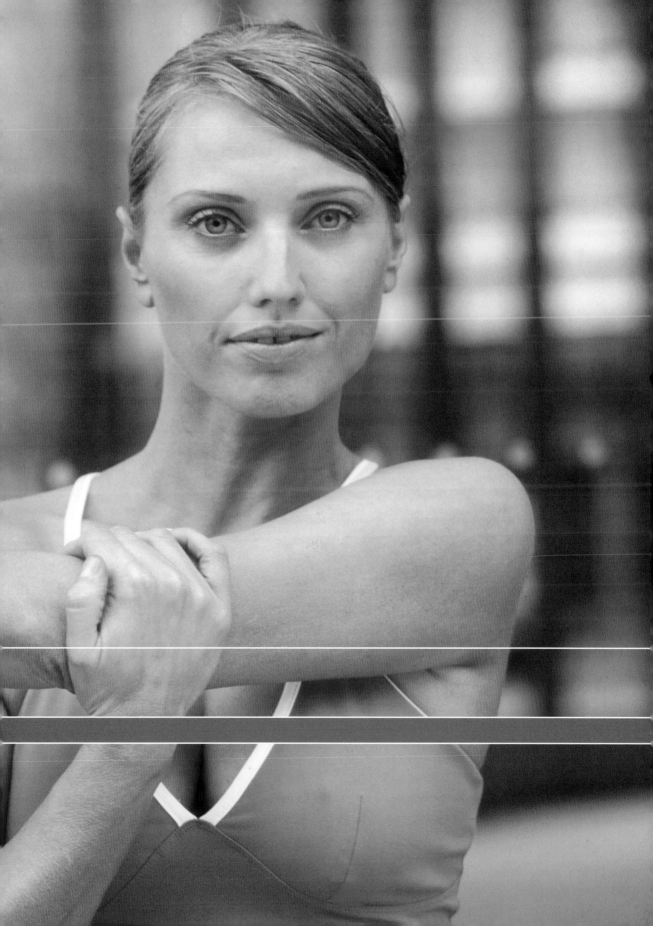

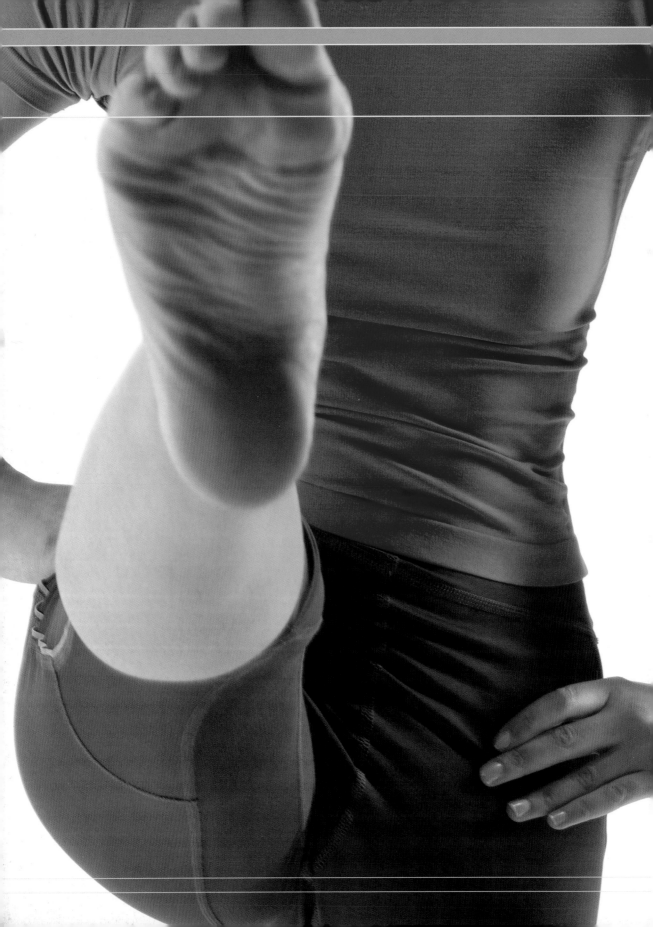

01

week 01

box press
abdominal crunch
lunge and kick

Here's where the new you begins. Turn the page and take your first steps on the road to becoming toned, fit and feeling great. The Week 01 toning exercises of the No-Gym Workout are straightforward moves to help you get started on your journey towards lasting health. Don't forget to do each exercise three times during the week.

box press
week 01 • upper body

This adapted press-up is a particularly good exercise for women as it doesn't require abs of steel just to maintain the starting position. Kneeling in the 'box' position and pulling in your abdominals empowers your arms and shoulders to push against your body weight, toning every major muscle group and giving you great upper-arm definition and upper-body strength.

WHAT DOES IT DO?

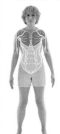

Tones the pectoral muscles (chest), the deltoids and triceps (arms) and the abdominals (stomach).

calories burned	5
weekly calories	15

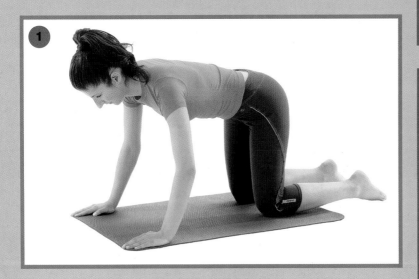

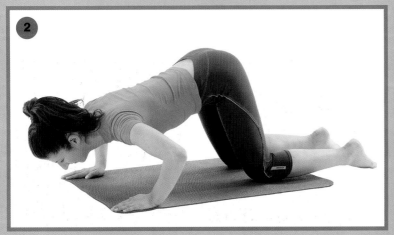

the exercise

1 Kneel on the floor with your knees directly under your hips. Your hands should be slightly wider than shoulder width apart. Keep your fingers pointing forwards, and check that your body weight is over your hands. Pull your tummy in tight, and keep your back flat. Imagine a straight line from your hips to your head keeping your body in alignment.

2 Breathe out as you lower your body, bending your arms so that your elbows make a 90-degree angle. Now inhale as you push back up to the starting position.

repeat 12–20x

O1

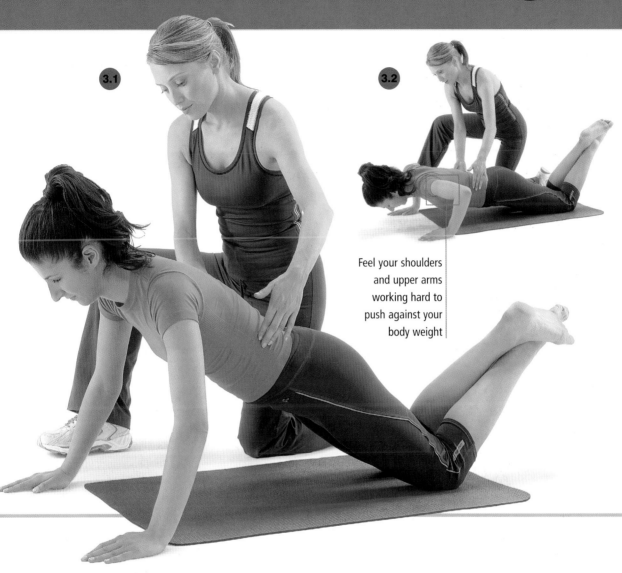

3.1

3.2

Feel your shoulders
and upper arms
working hard to
push against your
body weight

boost the burn

3 Do a three-quarter press up by moving your knees further down the mat, making an elongated box shape with your feet crossed. This position shifts more body weight onto your arms and shoulders, creating more resistance for your muscles. Work with a friend to check your position.

repeat 12–20x

what to avoid

Avoid arching your back and/or relaxing your abdominal muscles, letting your stomach sag. You need to pull in your abdominals to stay balanced and support your upper body as you move.

abdominal crunch
week 01 • middle body

The abdominal crunch is one of the most basic yet highly effective exercises, as it targets all the abdominal muscles helping you to work towards that hourglass shape by firming the stomach, defining the waist and strengthening and protecting the lower back. If you have back or neck problems, practise this exercise with your arms supporting your neck as shown in the variation.

WHAT DOES IT DO?

Tones the transversus abdominis, rectus abdominis and external oblique muscles of the stomach.

calories burned	3
weekly calories	9

1

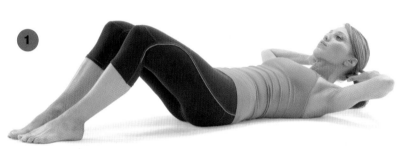

2

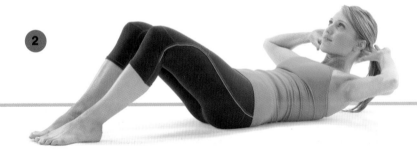

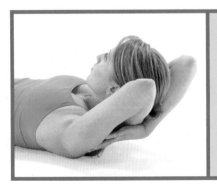

variation

If you suffer from back or neck problems, or feel any discomfort while practising this exercise, cross your arms behind your head, with your hands on the tops of your shoulders, to give support.

the exercise

1 Lie on your back with your knees up, making a right angle with the floor. Position your feet slightly apart. With your elbows out to the side, place your fingertips by your ears. Breathe in.

2 Engage your abdominal muscles and focus on moving from your stomach as you lift your head and shoulders off the floor as far as you can towards your knees. Exhale gently.

repeat 12–20x

3

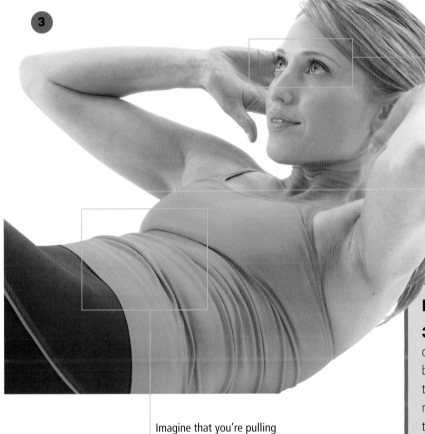

Focus just above the tops of your knees

Imagine that you're pulling your navel tight to your spine

boost the burn

3 Begin the crunch 2–3cm (1in) or so off the floor and raise your body a little higher. Don't be tempted to go too fast – the real benefit in this exercise is to progress slowly, which works the muscles more deeply.

repeat 12–20x

what to avoid

Pulling on your neck or head can cause injury and often means you're not using your abdominal muscles. It can be easy to fall into this trap when you're getting tired. If this is the case, stop, breathe for 10 seconds, then resume your reps.

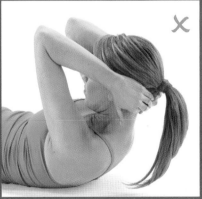

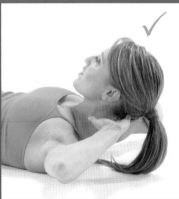

lunge and kick
week 01 • lower body

This move gets you thinner thighs, a firmer bottom and better balance, posture and alignment, as well as increasing your metabolic rate so you'll burn calories while you exercise and later when you rest. This is all because the lunge and kick tones the two largest muscles in your body – the quadriceps (leg) and gluteus maximus (buttocks), giving both the standing and supporting leg an even, simultaneous workout.

WHAT DOES IT DO?

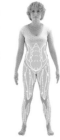

Tones the quadriceps and hamstrings (leg), gluteus maximus (buttocks), transversus abdominis (stomach) and gastrocnemius (calf muscles).

calories burned	14
weekly calories	42

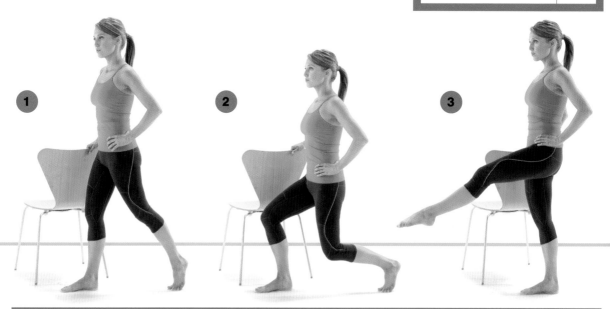

the exercise

1 Begin by standing with your right leg 30cm (1ft) or so in front of your left leg. Hold onto a chair for balance. Now check your posture, making sure you keep your back straight, shoulders down and draw in your stomach – imagine that your navel is touching your spine.

2 Maintaining this position, bend your knees until the lower part of your left leg is parallel to the floor, using the chair for support as you come lower down. Hold for two seconds.

3 Rise, bringing your left knee to a comfortable height, and kick forwards with pointed toes. Kick as high as is comfortable without leaning backwards, and return to the starting position. Breathe evenly throughout the exercise.

repeat 12–20x

01

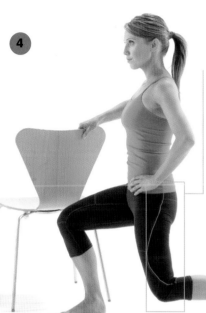

4

Keep your
knee in line
with your hip

5

Keep your
abdominals
pulled in tight

boost the burn

4 Begin in the starting position
shown in Step 1, but this time
lunge more deeply so that your
knee is positioned 5cm (2in) or
so off the floor.

5 Kick no higher that hip height
– the benefit is in the extra
intensity you'll feel in your thigh
muscles in the deeper lunge.
Stay aware of your posture,
keeping your shoulders back
and squeeze your buttocks tight.
You should feel your weight
through your heels.

repeat 12–20x

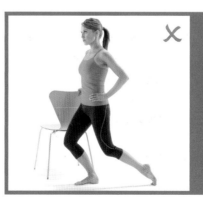

✗

what to avoid

Make sure that your knees don't
go forward of your toes – keep your
body weight back with your knee
aligned over your toes. Make sure
you always keep your stomach
pulled in to support your back.

case study • Ella

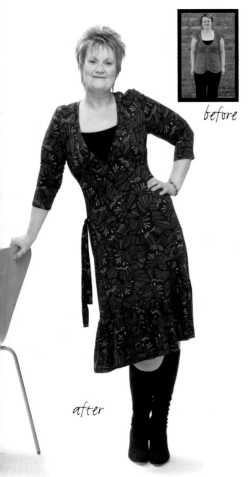

before

after

Name: Ella
Age: 47
Lifestyle: Living with partner, two grown-up children. Works full time as an administrator, so spends a lot of time seated at a desk.

'A few years ago I was 107kg (17 stone). I felt stiff, was tired all the time, and had high blood pressure – and at a size 20 or 22, I didn't feel much like socialising,' Ella begins. With Weightwatchers™, Ella began an amazing journey towards better health as she lost a total of 31.5kg (5 stone), dropped to a dress size 14 – and got her blood pressure back to normal.

She chose the No-Gym Workout after achieving her weight loss because she wanted to tone up and banish some of the loose skin around her arms and midriff. 'I felt I needed to lose a certain amount of weight first to be comfortable exercising,' Ella explains. 'I had never joined a gym before, because of my size.' Using a diary to record her maintenance diet and exercise helped her get started on the No-Gym Workout, and in six weeks, although weight loss was not her first priority, Ella lost 3kg (7lb).

'I fitted the workout in around work, setting aside an hour or so each day when I'd power walk or tone.' The variety of the exercises fired her motivation – 'every week the exercises change so you don't get bored' – and

Ella embraced the power walking with remarkable ease. 'I enjoyed the walking. It helped me to relax – I have six bosses and constant deadlines at work. I made a few friends walking my circuit, too. I began to see that

'I fitted the workout in around work, setting aside an hour or so each day, when I'd power walk or tone'

there was a whole world of people exercising and enjoying it, something I hadn't been aware of before.'

Soon, Ella began to see the results as she lost more weight on her arms, face and thighs, and the muscle tone in her upper arms improved. She also carried hand weights while power walking, which burns more calories (see page 36), and speeds toning. 'Now, I'm fitter, slimmer, happier with myself, and certainly more confident,' she concludes. 'In fact, I'm nearly into a size 12 jeans. I've kept a big tent dress that I used to wear as a reminder of just how far I've come!'

the results

Centimetre/inch loss after six weeks:

Bust: **3.75cm (1½in)**
Waist: **5cm (2in)**
Hips: **2.5cm (1in)**
Thighs: **5cm (2in)**
Knees: **2.5cm (1in)**
Upper arms: **3.75cm (1½in)**

questions and answers

I find it hard to find the time to exercise. What can I do?

This is a problem so many of us have! My solution is to make time in your day for Me Time, in addition to Car Time, Family Time, Work Time, Shopping Time and Telly Time. You need only find five minutes to do your toning exercises, and you can squeeze power walks into 20 minutes of your lunch hour. You'll feel the benefits for the rest of the day.

Is it better to use my own body weight for resistance during exercises or should I use fixed weight machines at the gym?

Without a doubt, it's far better to use your own body weight, because in doing so you engage lots of different muscles which must work together to stabilise the body. For example, when doing abdominal crunches (see pages 50–1) you use your body weight to tone the abdomen. This will mean you use (and tone) many abdominal muscles at the same time. Fixed weight machines, however, tend to isolate one muscle group, so the muscle worked is specific to that machine. Therefore, using a fixed weight machine means

you don't tone as many muscles as when you use your body weight for resistance. So your body is like a multi-gym that goes everywhere with you.

Should I exercise on an empty stomach?

No – you need fuel before exercise (see pages 40–1). If you exercise early in the day, a banana and a small glass of milk will give you energy. If you work out later in the day, be sure to have a small snack 30 minutes before you exercise.

What is the best way to get a flat tummy?

Abdominal crunches and rolls (see pages 50–1 and 98–9) will help. However, with any abdominal exercise, the key factor is technique. You need to engage the deepest abdominal muscle, the transversus abdominis. The name of the muscle may sound complicated, but it is very easy to activate – you simply pull in your belly button tight to the spine. So when doing your basic abdominal crunch, for example, always focus on pulling your navel in to the spine. As long as you engage this muscle when practising abdominal exercises, you will be working the entire abdominal muscle group, which gives you an extremely effective workout.

Is it better to perform the toning exercises quickly so I can do more repetitions?

I always say to my clients that quality is far more important than quantity. When you perform the exercises more slowly it's more challenging, so you get better results. You'll also begin to gain more control over your body, which feels satisfying. When you perform exercises too quickly, you encourage momentum and can cause potential injury. Always work slowly, and as you work think how your muscles are feeling at each stage of the movement. As you progress, you'll notice how your muscles begin to feel more powerful.

I'm new to exercise. How do I stop my muscles from hurting the next day?

Always do warm-up stretches before you begin walking and toning exercises (see pages 32–3), and hold the stretches for a few seconds longer than recommended. Also, don't do toning exercises on two or more consecutive days, because you can strain your muscles this way – you need a day's recovery (see page 18) so this is why you power walk on the alternate days instead of toning.

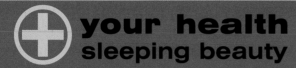 your health
sleeping beauty

By exercising this week, you've just improved your sleep patterns and you will be enjoying more deep, restorative REM sleep, which regenerates muscles, rejuvenates cells, gives you the energy to exercise and keeps you looking younger for longer.

Sleep problems are more commonplace than you'd imagine – more than one million people in Britain now take prescription sleeping pills. However, exercising regularly can dramatically improve your sleep experience without the need to reach for the bottle. Research has shown that exercise promotes the production of the hormone melatonin, secreted by the pineal gland in the brain's hypothalamus. Melatonin regulates your internal body clock, or circadian rhythms, so that you feel naturally sleepy at night and alert during daylight hours. As more melatonin circulates through your system, your body's sleep-wake cycles become stronger – so with increased exercise each week, you'll get to sleep more easily, and suffer less from restlessness or wakefulness during the night.

Exercise not only improves sleep patterns, but can radically improve sleep quality, which affects how you function throughout the day. When you're fit and active, you naturally get more REM (rapid eye movement) sleep – this is sleep during which you are deeply relaxed and dreaming dreams that you remember, as opposed to non-REM sleep.

Although your body needs both types of sleep, the more REM sleep you get, the better, because during REM sleep, human growth hormone is released which rejuvenates and repairs the body's cells, keeping you healthy and young-looking. Studies have shown that some athletes spend up to one hour longer in REM sleep than non-athletes.

However, you don't need more sleep because you're exercising – you can sleep for the same number of hours as usual but literally get more out of it because your body spends proportionally longer in a REM state than a non-REM state, producing more human growth hormone. Your body repairs itself – and you wake up feeing relaxed and refreshed, rather than tired and disorientated

how many hours a night?

Sleep needs vary from person to person, but health professionals recommend around eight hours a night. Some studies also suggest that women need to sleep for an hour longer than men.

ways to sleep easy

• Eat foods containing the amino acid tryptophan, a sleep-inducer. These include cottage cheese, bananas, turkey and, strangely, lettuce, which contains the natural sedative lacturcarium.
• Snack on light carbohydrates, such as a small slice of wholemeal bread, before going to bed.
• Get the mineral balance right. Calcium and magnesium are needed for good sleep, hence warm milk and honey has endured as the perfect bedtime drink. The milk provides calcium and the honey is a good source of magnesium.

SLEEP TO LOSE WEIGHT

Recent studies have shown that if you're sleep deprived, you're less likely to lose weight. Lack of sleep affects the hormones that control appetite, making you hungry. Studies have shown that, on average, people who are overweight are those who tend to get the least amount of sleep.

01

• Go to bed earlier, particularly if you're feeling stressed out. Anxiety and prolonged periods of stress send your adrenal glands into overdrive and exhaustion. The earlier you go to bed before 12 o'clock, the better – sleep before midnight helps to restore the adrenal glands more effectively than sleep after midnight.

what to avoid

• Caffeine late in the day – substitute your luscious after-dinner latte for a virtuous peppermint or ginger tea (good for digestion) or soothing camomile.
• Monosodium glutamate (MSG), found in many prepared meals and some Eastern-style foods, which can interfere with sleep.
• Spicy foods, which stimulate rather than relax the body.
• A heavy, rich meal high in protein and carbs – this can have your digestive system working overtime, late into the night, and keep you uncomfortably awake.
• Too much alcohol – a little nightcap is fine as it will usually make you feel drowsy, but too many alcoholic drinks in the evening cause dehydration and sleep disturbance often in the early hours of the morning.
• The 'guilt' workout – when you've eaten too many of the wrong foods during the day and decide to go for an evening workout to burn it off. Ideally you should finish exercising four hours or more before bedtime, or the adrenaline rush you get from exercising will keep you awake.

little extras

• Lavender essential oil has a soporific effect – add about six drops to a warm bath after you've run the water.
• The herb valerian helps sleep and can be found commercially as Valerina™.
• Melatonin is available as a supplement outside the UK, and is effective at regulating sleep. Many travellers purchase it in the USA and use it to alleviate the symptoms of jet lag.

record your progress

Fill in the blanks below to chart your success.

Measurements before the start of Week 01:	Measurements at the end of Week 01:
bust	bust
waist	waist
hips	hips
thighs	thighs
upper arms	upper arms

How many power walks did you do?

1 2 3 4

How many pedometer steps?

How many toning sessions did you do?

1 2 3 4

Rate your healthy eating this week

1 2 3 4 5 (1, poor and 5, excellent)

Rate your water intake this week

1 2 3 4 5 (1, poor and 5, excellent)

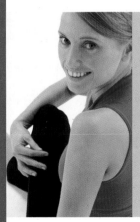

'Well done, you have completed your first week and already you will have increased your metabolism and started to tone up.'

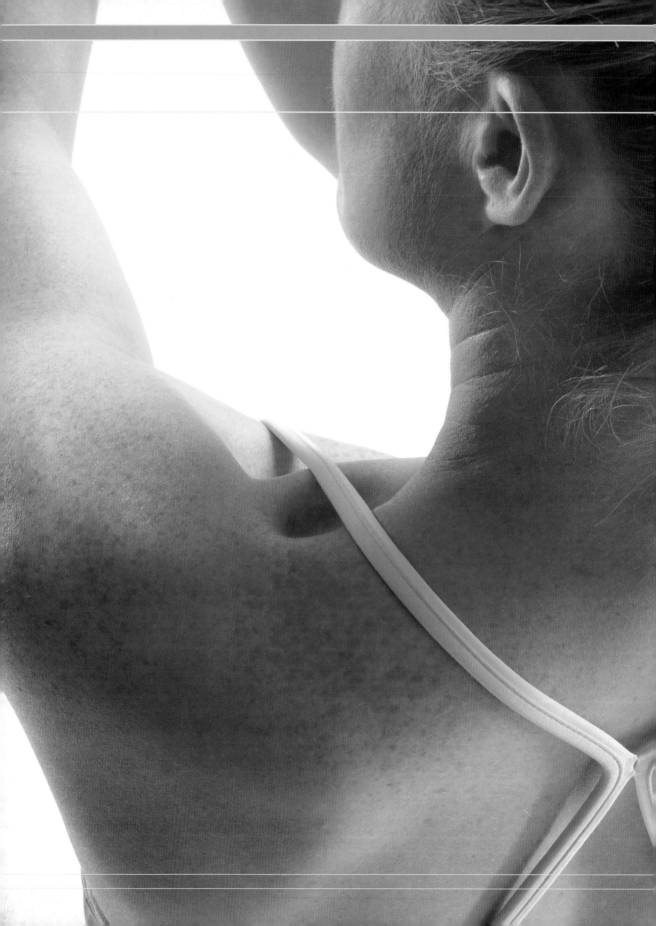

02

week 02

elbow and bust press
standing oblique twist
wide-leg squat

With your first week completed you will already have improved your health and naturally increased your metabolism. As you start to feel re-energised, don't be afraid of your tape measure – be proud of the changes it reveals, no matter how small.

elbow and bust press
week 02 • upper body

This exercise is practically a surgery-saver – it helps to draw and lift the muscle and deep fibrous tissue that supports the bust and tones the back of the upper arms, and is therefore a particularly great move for those areas that are beginning to give in to gravity.

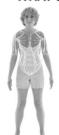

WHAT DOES IT DO?

The elbow and bust press works five major muscles, toning the pectoralis major (chest), shoulders, triceps, biceps and abdominals.

calories burned	4
weekly calories	12

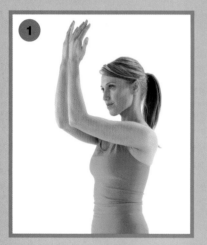

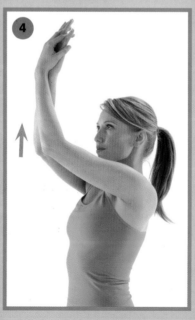

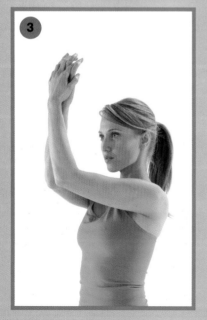

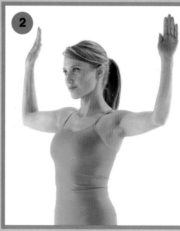

the exercise

Begin by standing with your feet hip-width apart, and keep your knees soft. Pull in your abdominal muscles.

1 Bring your elbows up to shoulder height, so your wrists are about the same level as the crown of your head.

2 Bring your arms out to the side, then back to the centre, for eight repetitions.

3 Now squeeze your forearms together and interlace your fingers.

4 Lift up your arms towards the ceiling, then lower your elbows to shoulder height, keeping your forearms squeezed together.

repeat 12–20x

02

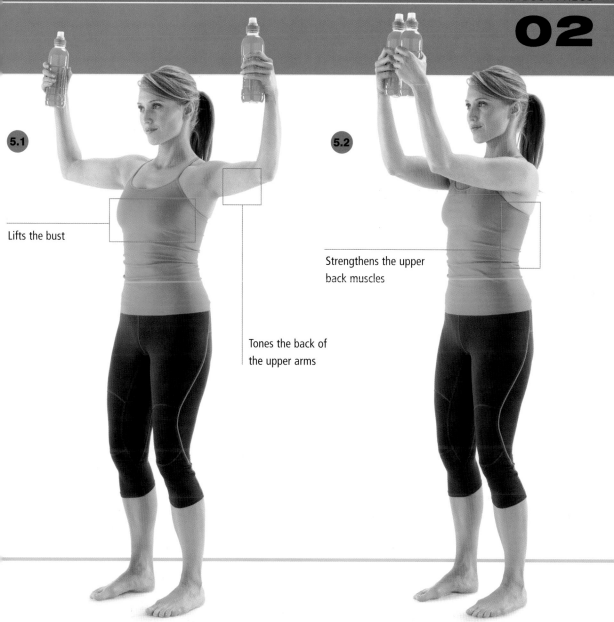

5.1

Lifts the bust

Tones the back of
the upper arms

5.2

Strengthens the upper
back muscles

boost the burn

5 Practise the first move, taking your arms out to the side, while holding
two small bottles of water – begin with filling them a third full, topping up
the water level as you get stronger and need more resistance. Hold one or
both bottles while doing the lifting action with your forearms clasped.

repeat 12–20x

what to avoid

Keep your elbows together – it's
easy to let them drift apart. Check
your arm position, too – don't let
your arms drop too low. If this
happens, pull in your abdominals
to correct your posture.

standing oblique twist
week 02 • middle body

The standing twist draws in the waist and tones the transverse abdominal muscle – the deepest stomach muscle – enabling you to tone your stomach without getting down on the floor for crunches. It's also great for improving posture, so practise this exercise if you're prone to slouching.

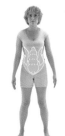

WHAT DOES IT DO?

Tones the oblique muscles, which criss-cross your waist, and the transversus abdominis muscle.

calories burned	8
weekly calories	24

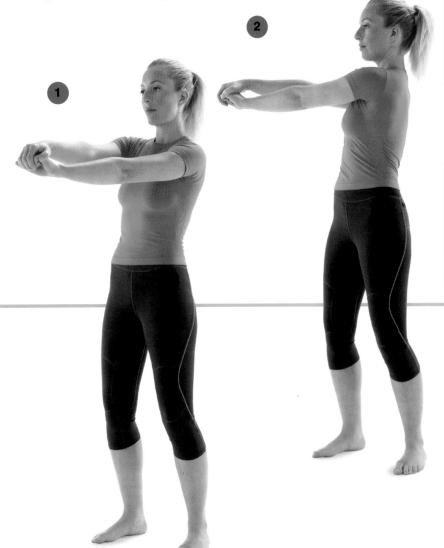

the exercise

1 Stand with your feet hip-width apart, with your knees soft and your arms extended in front of you and your hands clasped, one on top of the other. Keep your shoulders, back and neck relaxed.

2 Keeping your hips facing forwards, breathe in then exhale as you slowly rotate your upper body and arms as far to the side as you can. Pull in your abdominal muscles and feel your body weight settle in your hips. Return to the centre, then repeat the exercise on the opposite side.

repeat 12–20x

02

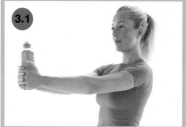

3.1

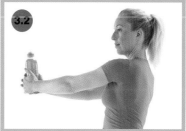

3.2

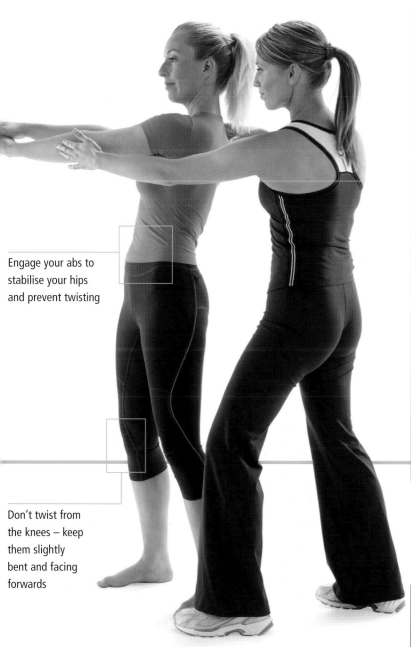

Engage your abs to stabilise your hips and prevent twisting

Don't twist from the knees – keep them slightly bent and facing forwards

boost the burn

3 Use a full bottle of water, a hand weight or a resistance band to intensify the workout in the arms and in the oblique muscles of the waist.

repeat 12–20x

what to avoid

Don't lock your knees.

Don't let your hips swivel – keep your pelvis pointing forwards.

wide-leg squat
week 02 • lower body

This amazing exercise works practically the entire lower body in one simple move. Ballerinas practise it to build strength in their legs and improve posture. It elongates the leg muscles, so this is the perfect pose if you want thinner thighs, and it also tightens the buttock muscles to give you that J-Lo lift.

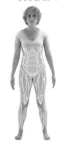

WHAT DOES IT DO?

The wide-leg squat works eight major muscle groups, toning the quadriceps, bottom, hamstrings, inner thighs, outer thighs, hips, calves and abdominals.

calories burned	9
weekly calories	27

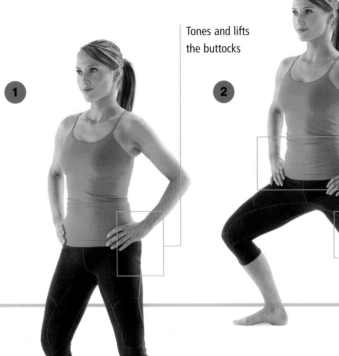

Tones and lifts the buttocks

Works the abdominal muscles, toning the middle body

Tones the inner and outer thighs

the exercise

1 Stand with your feet slightly wider than shoulder-width apart. Bend your knees and turn your toes out diagonally. Keeping your upper body perfectly straight and with your hands on your hips, pull in your abdominal muscles.

2 Slowly bend through your knees so your thighs are as close to horizontal as possible. Keep your bottom squeezed tight as you hold in your abdominal muscles. Count to five, then straighten.

repeat 12–20x

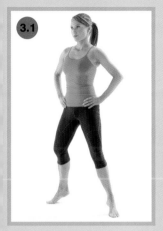

3.1

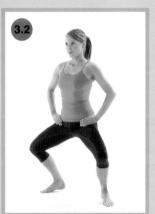

3.2

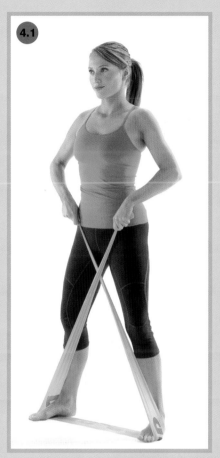

4.1

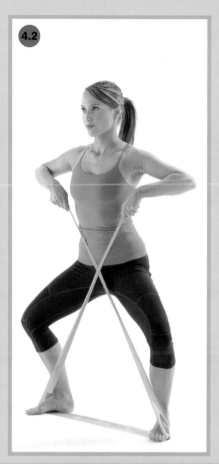

4.2

boost the burn

3 Begin in the starting position, with your hands on your hips. Raise both heels off the floor then repeat steps 1 and 2. The heel lift is great for toning the inner thighs and calf muscles.

4 You can use a resistance band crossed over your body as shown to increase resistance. Using the band also gives your arms a good workout. Keep both heels on the floor and repeat the regular move. You'll feel the muscles of your bottom and thighs working deeply.

repeat 12–20x

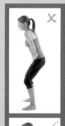

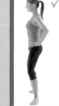

what to avoid

Don't lean forward because you lose the squeeze on your abdominal muscles. Equally, don't let your knees fall inward or drop your hips so that they are lower than your knees.

case study · Jessie

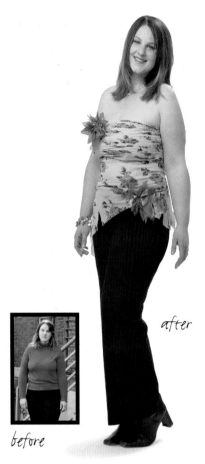

after

before

Name: Jessie
Age: 27
Lifestyle: Living with partner. Full-time probation officer; currently on maternity leave. Busy with newborn baby and three-and-a-half year old child.

'Ive been a yo-yo dieter all my life, probably lurching between a size 12 and a size 18,' Jessie explains. 'I've always done a sedentary job and never been sporty, so achieving my ideal size 12–14 has been a challenge.' Jessie tried the No-Gym Workout to lose weight and tone her stomach after having her second child, and it really has made a difference. 'What worked for me was that the exercises were do-able, and they fitted around the kids. I could power walk while pushing the pram and exercise at home while keeping an eye on them, which is something I'd never be able to do at the gym – I couldn't get there with a baby and a small child to look after.'

Jessie quickly noticed a difference in her energy levels and mood when she started exercising regularly. 'I found that I could use the exercise routine as a way to channel stress,' she says, and this in turn improved her energy levels as she began to enjoy the programme more than she had anticipated. 'I feel so much better – it has been great to get some abdominal strength back, and in addition I feel much more confident than I did before I started,' she smiles.

Jessie's watchword for her diet is moderation. She devised her own healthy eating plan based on cutting out a lot of sugar and fat from her diet. 'Watch your portion sizes,' she advises, 'and really think about whether or not you are full. Waiting for five minutes between courses to decide if I really was still hungry helped me stop over-eating.'

Another mental switch Jessie made was to see her new lifestyle as normal, not a diet, and her exercises just part of her usual routine. 'At the end of the six weeks I was down to a size 14–16,' she happily confides. 'I intend to keep going now so I can tone up and lose even more weight before I return to work.'

'what worked for me is that the exercises were do-able, and they fitted around the kids – I could power walk while pushing the pram and exercise at home'

the results

No measurements taken; preferred the scales.

Starting weight: **83kg (13st 2lb)**
After six weeks: **73kg (11st 9lb)**
Loss: **10kg (1st 7lb)**
Starting dress size: **16–18**
After six weeks: **14–16**

questions and answers

I'm worried that toning exercises will make my muscles bulk up. How can I stop this happening?

To build muscle bulk, you would have to push extremely heavy weights. You would also need to have the same testosterone level as a man – which is naturally impossible. So with the No-Gym Workout, be assured that you won't build muscle bulk – instead, you'll gain lean muscle and great definition where it counts, particularly on the upper arms and thighs.

What's the most effective way to burn off the fat around my waist and hips?

There's no single solution to stubborn fat in these areas – the answer is a combination of all three elements of this programme: toning exercises, power walking and consistent healthy eating. Within three weeks you'll notice a difference in your body shape, and you'll look and feel so much better than before.

Can I do my toning exercises every day?

No – rather than speed up results, toning every day could result in injury. Your muscles need 24 hours to recover from toning exercises. After exertion, muscles must rest to recover, repair and grow stronger. If you toned every day you would feel sore and tired all the time, which would also lower your motivation.

Will the No-Gym Workout get rid of my cellulite?

Cellulite – fatty deposits on the bottom and thighs – is the bane of some very slim women as well as those who are overweight, so the impact of exercise on cellulite can vary according to the individual. I advise my clients to follow the workout, drink plenty of water, cut down on caffeine and get into the habit of body-brushing in the shower twice a week. Use a specially designed brush and always brush towards the heart to boost the circulation and help break down fatty deposits.

What are your tips for keeping going with the programme and eating healthily without giving up?

The minute you start exercising, you start to feel good. Exercise encourages the release of endorphins, the body's happiness chemical. As your diet improves, you'll feel in better health, and mentally you'll gain confidence as you feel more in control of your lifestyle. So once you start, you won't want to stop.

I want to lose weight – would I not lose more weight running rather than power walking?

This is a good question, because throughout my years of fitness training I have always found that the clients who get the best results and maintain them are those who power walk, rather than those who run. The reason for this, I believe, is because these clients enjoy the walking so they stick to it. I also believe that walking is the best way to tone your bottom, thighs, arms and tummy while burning fat at the same time. Our bodies are designed to walk – if we were meant to run, we would have extra padding in our heels. The impact of running can cause damage to joints, so for this reason, power walking is also a safer way to exercise.

How will working on my quadriceps, bottom, back and chest help me to lose weight?

Your quadriceps, chest, back and bottom contain your largest muscles. They have the most muscle fibres, and therefore burn more calories than other smaller muscles. If your goal is to lose weight, you need to tone these muscles so that your body naturally burns more calories.

✚ your health
preventing osteoporosis

By exercising this week, you've just given yourself added protection against the bone-thinning disease osteoporosis. This can affect post-menopausal women and is a serious condition. However, you can take steps to decrease your chances of getting osteoporosis by following the No-Gym Workout, or by doing other regular exercise, during your thirties, forties and beyond to help your body build vital bone mass and bone density that is necessary to keep you strong and healthy.

It's thought that about three million people in the UK suffer from osteoporosis – when bone mass and bone density decrease, causing bones to become weak and increasing the risk of fractures. Osteoporosis affects more women than men (although men do suffer from the disease) because low levels of the hormone oestrogen can reduce bone mass and bone density. Post-menopausal women are therefore at risk, as their oestrogen levels will naturally decrease after menopause. Oestrogen supports bone mass and density, so bones can become weak, brittle and prone to fracture.

Unfortuantely, many women don't realise they have osteoporosis until they suffer a fracture – the hips, legs, arms and shoulders are particularly vulnerable. The good news, however, is that bone scans can diagnose onset, measuring the mineral density in bones, which indicates if they are becoming weakened and brittle. If you think you are at risk, ask your doctor about bone scans.

Osteoporosis is usually treated by hormone replacement therapy and by taking calcium and vitamin D supplements – vitamin D promotes the absorption of calcium. Exposure to the sun for 10 or 15 minutes a day fires the body into vitamin D production, but older people and those living in colder countries with little sunshine usually don't get enough vitamin D this way. Prevention is, of course, infinitely preferable – and one of the best ways to protect yourself from osteoporosis is by exercising.

are you at risk?

If any of the following describes your past or present health issues or lifestyle, you may be at risk.

• If you are thin or underweight you may tend to have lower bone mass and bone density than people who are of an average weight.

• If you have suffered from the eating disorder anorexia, which interferes with the menstrual cycle and causes lowered oestrogen levels.

• If you exercise excessively, which can cause a drop in oestrogen, the bone-helping hormone.

• If you have a very inactive lifestyle – exercise keeps bones healthy.

• If you smoke – a study in the *Journal of the American Academy of Orthopedic Surgeons* (2001) shows that smoking depletes the health of muscles, bones and joints. For women, the nicotine in cigarettes also brings down oestrogen levels, reducing bone mass.

• If you don't have enough calcium in your diet (see the nutrition tips, right, on topping up your calcium intake).

• If you are very stressed – this encourages high levels of the hormone cortisone, which can break down bone tissue.

• If you cannot absorb nutrients well because you have digestive disorders such as Crohn's disease, colitis or coeliac disease.

• If you are deficient in vitamin D, which supports bone health.

• If you have a family history of osteoporosis.

NUTRITION TIPS

Whenever possible, avoid excessive amounts of acid-forming food and drink. Your body is naturally slightly alkaline, so to compensate for excess acid, it excretes calcium from the bones, which has an alkaline effect. Non-herbal teas, coffee and carbonated drinks in particular are acid-forming, as are meat, refined carbohydrates and sugar.

Keep your calcium levels up – the government's RDA (recommended daily allowance) is 800mg of calcium a day. Find it in tinned fish such as sardines, leafy green vegetables, sesame seeds, pulses, nuts and milk and cheese (stick to lower-fat varieties).

You can, however, significantly reduce your osteoporosis risk at any time by exercising regularly and eating well. It doesn't matter if you've never exercised until now – the important thing is that you have begun. You can improve your health at any age – you're never too old to start an exercise programme.

how does exercise help?

Doing weight-bearing or resistance exercise builds bone mass and bone density. When you push against your own body weight – when doing a press-up, for example – the action causes the muscles to rub against the bone. This stimulates the production of a substance called matrix. Matrix supports bone mass and bone density – it therefore follows that the more you do this kind of exercise, the stronger your bones will be.

Regular exercise also improves posture and balance, which in turn helps to prevent potential falls in older people whose bones naturally become more brittle with age.

record your progress

Fill in the blanks below to chart your success.

Measurements before the start of Week 02:	Measurements at the end of Week 02:
bust	bust
waist	waist
hips	hips
thighs	thighs
upper arms	upper arms

How many power walks did you do?

1   2   3   4

How many pedometer steps?

How many toning sessions did you do?

1   2   3   4

Rate your healthy eating this week

1   2   3   4   5   (1, poor and 5, excellent)

Rate your water intake this week

1   2   3   4   5   (1, poor and 5, excellent)

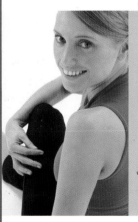

'The body reacts quickly to exercise and a healthy lifestyle – you will be feeling fitter and your body shape is starting to change.'

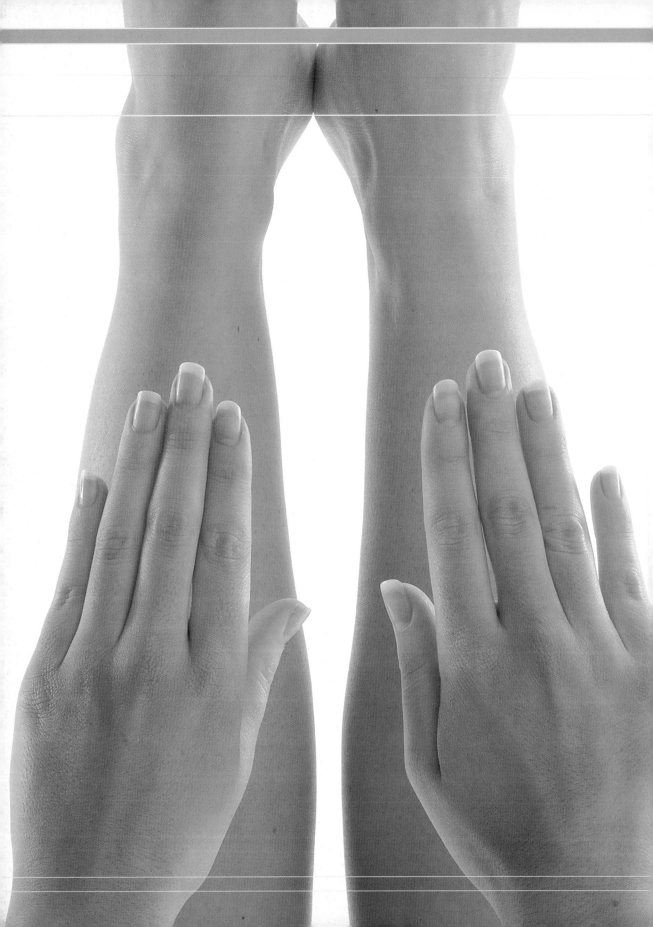

week 03

overhead arm press
toe reaches
hamstring kicks

By the end of this week you are halfway through the programme and it's time to start seeing the results. You will have more lean muscle and your clothes will be feeling looser. If you are feeling this good after only three weeks, just imagine how you will feel after six!

overhead arm press
week 03 • upper body

The arm press works out the major muscles in the entire upper body and improves the range of movement in your back, shoulders and arms. You'll also use your abdominal muscles to maintain your posture as you work your arms, which will support your back and firm your core muscles.

WHAT DOES IT DO?

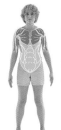

Tones the latissimus dorsi muscles of the back as well as the shoulder, arm and abdominal muscles.

calories burned	5
weekly calories	15

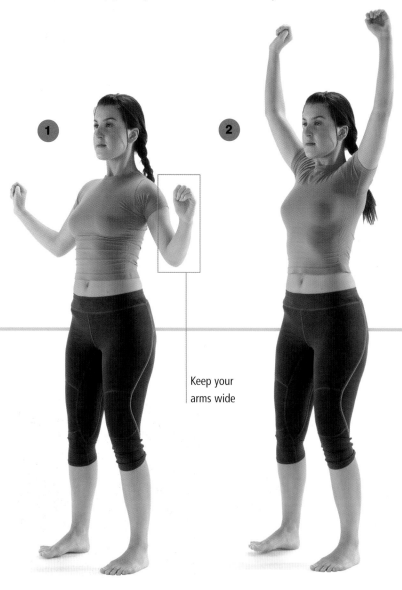

1

2

Keep your arms wide

the exercise

1 Stand with your feet hip-width apart and your knees slightly bent. Bend your arms and raise your elbows to shoulder height. Breathe in.

2 Breathe out as you slowly raise your arms over your head, straightening them until your elbows are extended but not locked. Keeping your abdominal muscles pulled in, feel the muscles working in your arms, chest and back. Slowly return to the starting position.

repeat 12–20x

03

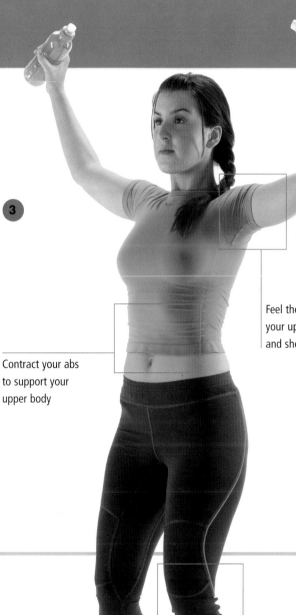

3

boost the burn

3 Repeat the exercise using filled water bottles or hand weights. This contracts the muscles more deeply making them work harder.

repeat 12–20x

Feel the burn in your upper arms and shoulders

Contract your abs to support your upper body

Keep your weight through the backs of your legs and heels

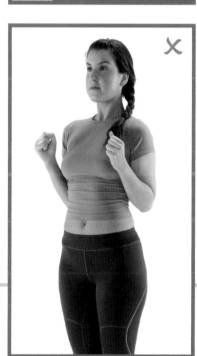

what to avoid

Don't let your arm position narrow, as you'll lose intensity. Keep the movement wide throughout the exercise and don't lock your knees.

toe reaches
week 03 • middle body

This exercise is a fantastic leg and stomach toner, targeting those key areas which, when toned, can change the whole way you dress. It looks deceptively simple, but you'll be flexing the hamstrings and toning the abdominal muscles, giving you an intense workout and, with practice, a taut midriff and toned, supple thighs.

WHAT DOES IT DO?

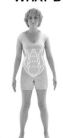

Tones the abdominal muscles – the rectus abdominis, the transversus abdominis and the obliques.

calories burned	3
weekly calories	9

1

Squeeze your thighs and bottom tightly to tone and stretch the hamstrings

Don't pull your head – rest your fingers at the top of your neck

2

the exercise

1 Lie on your back and raise your legs to form a 90-degree angle with the floor. Breathe in and exhale gradually as you pull your navel tight to your spine and slowly lift your hands up towards your toes. Lift your head and shoulders off the floor.

2 Reach up as high as you can, aiming for your toes, keeping your arms straight. Release.

repeat 12–20x

03

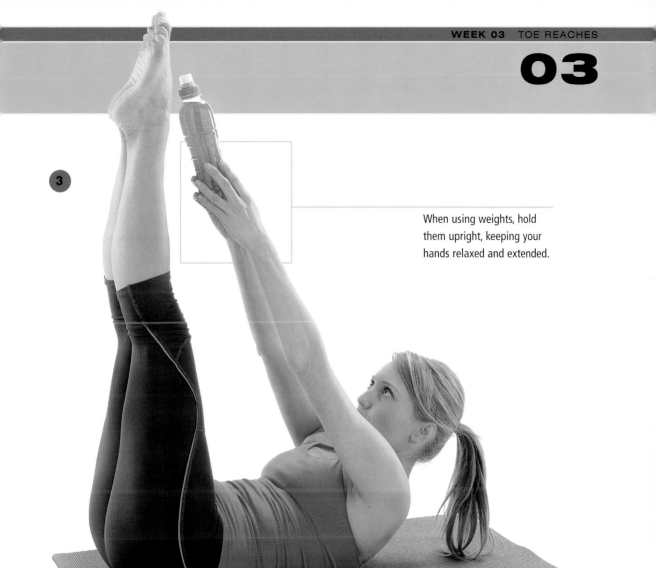

3

When using weights, hold
them upright, keeping your
hands relaxed and extended.

boost the burn

3 Perform the basic exercise, but
hold a hand weight or a bottle
filled with water. Hold your weight
steady and upright as you move.

repeat 12–20x

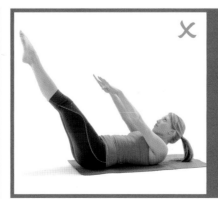

what to avoid

Make sure that your legs are
always over your hips to avoid
strain on your back – don't let your
legs veer away from you towards
the floor as this puts pressure on
your back and takes the focus off
the abs. Don't let your back arch.

hamstring kicks
week 03 • lower body

The kick is the ultimate hip and thigh shaper. The kicking action improves hamstring flexibility and works the hip and buttock muscles, but the challenge in this exercise is achieving an absolutely smooth kicking action and changeover to the opposite leg – you will need to engage your abdominal muscles at all times for complete control. You'll also benefit from better upper-body posture.

WHAT DOES IT DO?

Works the hamstrings and the gluteus maximus (hip/buttock) muscle of the working leg, the abdominals and all the muscles of the standing leg.

calories burned	9
weekly calories	27

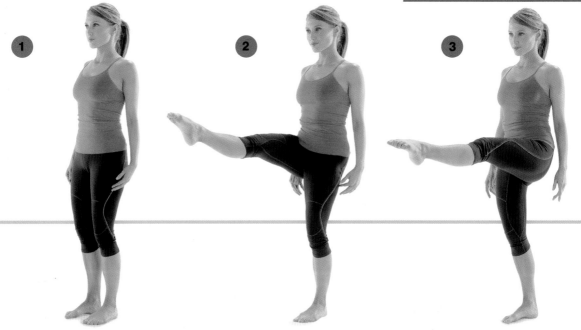

the exercise

1 Stand with your feet slightly apart and your arms down by your sides. Check that your knees are soft and your shoulders are back. Imagine that you are pulling in your navel tight to your spine. Hold in your stomach. Breathe evenly.

2 Make a controlled kick forward and back, without leaning forward.

Support your lower back by keeping your abdominal muscles firm.

3 Repeat the exercise on the opposite leg.

repeat 12–20x

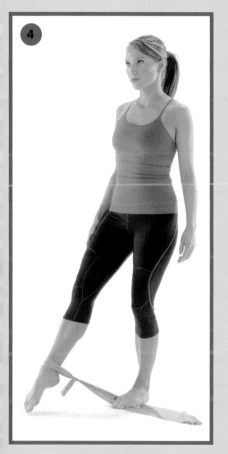

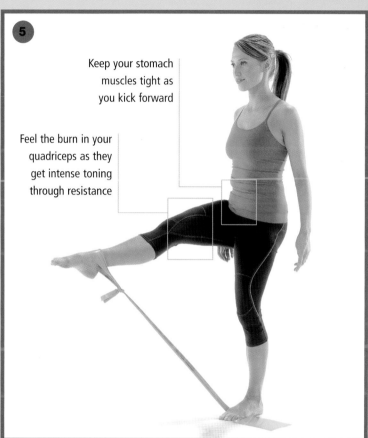

Keep your stomach muscles tight as you kick forward

Feel the burn in your quadriceps as they get intense toning through resistance

boost the burn

4 Use a resistance band knotted to your kicking leg. Stand on the other end with your standing leg. The band creates more resistance and makes the thigh muscles of the kicking leg work harder.

5 Keep your abdominals pulled in as you lift your leg and kick.

repeat 12–20x

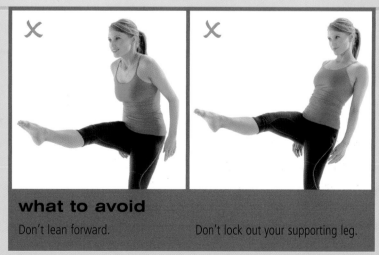

what to avoid

Don't lean forward.   Don't lock out your supporting leg.

case study · Emma

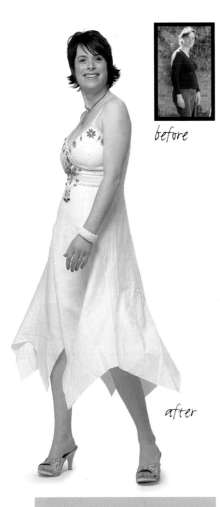

before

after

the results

No measurements taken. However, Emma dropped a dress size to a small size 12 or size 10. Her clothes feel looser and she has noticed the weight loss, in particular around her waist and hips.

Name: Emma
Age: 37
Lifestyle: Married. Full-time mother of three children aged five, three and one.

Emma used to be able to eat pretty much anything she wanted without worrying about her figure, but after she had her children she started putting on weight. 'I found myself comfort eating, usually going for the children's biscuits. Although I did lose weight through breastfeeding, later on I gained a few pounds. But what bothered me more was that my muscle tone was so poor. I couldn't even hold my stomach in.'

Emma decided to combat her sweet tooth with low GI (glycaemic index) foods such as wholegrain bread, rice, fruits and vegetables, and to tackle her lack of muscle tone with the No-Gym Workout.

'Getting to the gym would have been impossible for me, but what I liked about Lucy's programme was that the exercises were so simple. And I could feel them working early on.' As well as firming her stomach and bottom ('For the first time since having the children, I didn't mind the sight of my bottom in the mirror,' she says), Emma got a real buzz out of the power walks. 'This part of the programme was great,' she says, and, like many of the other case studies

in this book, Emma has decided to continue power walking and make it a part of her everyday routine.

Emma suffers from PCOS (polycystic ovary syndrome), a hormone condition that has a number of symptoms, including weight gain and fertility problems. Exercise is recommended because it helps to control the weight gain associated with the condition. Although Emma

'what I liked about Lucy's programme was that the exercises were so simple — and I could feel them working'

has not experienced excessive weight gain due to PCOS, building muscle tone and getting fitter will help to safeguard her health for the future.

So what kept Emma motivated? 'I realised that lapses don't matter, as long as you pick it up again. You don't have to be perfect — it's hard sticking to a plan when you've got a busy lifestyle. I'm just happy that I've found some exercises that are manageable and that I enjoy.'

questions and answers

When is the best time to train?

It's best to train when your body is warm. A warm body means your muscles are more pliable and facilitate a bigger range of movement – and you are least likely to injure yourself (see pages 32–3). Always warm up with a few stretches before toning and power walking. In terms of what time of day is best for you, personally, I think it's fine to train whenever it suits you – this is one of the great advantages of the No-Gym Workout. But do make it a priority to find time to tone and power walk.

How do I get rid of the spare tyre around my tummy?

It's not possible to spot-reduce fat. If a spare tyre is your main problem area, you'll still need a combination of power walking, sticking to a healthy eating plan and toning. The middle body exercises in the programme will tone your waist and abdominals and also boost your metabolic rate, so that you use more calories and burn off fat.

What exercise will get rid of my saddlebags?

Saddlebags – or the fat that collects around the tops of the thighs – can be difficult to banish, particularly if you're a natural pear shape (see pages 122–5). Your saddlebags will diminish as you reduce your overall body fat through toning and power walking, but you can't spot-reduce fat only on the thighs. The best approach is to do the exercises for pear shapes on page 124, which are designed to tone muscle around the hips and thighs, and give you definition as you work through the programme.

How much weight can I expect to lose on the No-Gym Workout?

It's important to remember that this workout is all about centimetre/inch loss and achieving a new, healthy you. However, a side-effect of the programme will be weight loss at a healthy and permanent level of between 450 and 900g (1–2lb) per week. Losing any more weight than this is drastic and only slows down your metabolism – which is why people who go on fad diets find their weight yo-yos. See the case studies on pages 54, 66, 78, 90, 102 and 114 – these women used their clothes, the scales and the tape measure to record their progress.

I'm 57 – does this make me too old to start exercising?

Absolutely not – you are never too old to exercise. One of my fittest clients is in her late sixties, and is super-fit and looks fantastic. She had a stroke and lost movement down the left side of her body, but through exercise she has made great progress towards recovery, regaining almost her full range of movement in her left arm and leg. She runs and can do press-ups. So there really is no excuse for being unfit. You should, however, always remember to check with your doctor before beginning any new exercise regime.

I eat healthily most of the time, but is it OK to splurge out once in a while – on a dessert or chocolate bar, for example?

Yes, you can have occasional treats but you do need to monitor how many and how often. It can sometimes feel as if you have few indulgences, particularly when you are radically changing your eating habits, but when you write them down and add them up at the end of a week, for example, it's likely that you're treating yourself more than you think. The best approach is to focus on being good 80 per cent of the time, so allow yourself the occasional chocolate bar when you really can't resist it. Just make sure you train for a little longer the following day and follow the diet tips on pages 20–3.

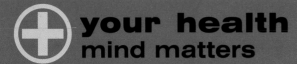

your health
mind matters

In the willpower culture of sport and fitness, the influence of our emotional patterns can often be neglected. We can be guilty of sabotaging our own efforts because it is easier to put other people first or because we lack confidence in ourselves. It's therefore vital to care for your emotions as you would care for your body – allow yourself time for goal-setting and make sure you reward your efforts.

Below are 10 simple ways to help you think positively. Try any one of these ideas when you need a boost – lack of motivation, not a lack of ability to succeed, is the major reason why most people fail at any given task. A positive mental attitude also benefits everyone around you, so share these ideas if you feel that they could help others.

1 Treat yourself Vow to reward yourself at the end of each week, whenever you've completed your three toning sessions and power walks (remember to fill in the checklists at the end of every week to monitor your progress). Allocate a reward jar and try to save a set amount of cash every day to pay for incentives such as a manicure. Alternatively, aim to save up a larger amount of money so that at the end of the six weeks you can buy a fabulous new outfit – in a smaller size.

2 Set achievable goals Don't paralyse yourself with pressure. Just set yourself one goal for each day – a power walk, or toning, or eating five portions of fruit and vegetables (see page 20–1). Achieve this, then move on to the next day's goals. If you don't succeed, don't beat yourself up. Move on to the next day and another goal that is achievable.

3 Visualise the way you want to look
Imagine yourself slim and fit. Make sure you do this every day, whenever you're having a quiet moment – for example, as you're about to check your emails, when you're washing

up or when you're about to go to sleep. Feed yourself with positive images and you'll quickly find your attitude becomes more positive.

4 Visualise letting go ... of resentment, guilt, anger or fear. See yourself placing these feelings in a bundle with wings and let them fly. Another effective visualisation is to imagine that you're breathing in light, and letting go of darkness. See your in-breath as light or white, and your exhalation as black, so you visualise breathing in goodness and breathing out negativity.

5 Maintain your self-belief Try not to focus on your failings – for example, if you've over-eaten or lapsed on the exercise programme. Don't beat yourself up: whenever you feel dispirited, take a note book and pen and write down five things that you've done in the last year which have made you feel proud or happy. Read them back to yourself as a reminder of how successful you have been, and can be.

6 Break the comfort-eating cycle Visualise a barrier between your hand and mouth, or better still, a lock on your fridge when you know you're about to eat because you're bored.

7 Take it easy Enjoy a body scrub (see opposite). Afterwards, run a hot bath, light some candles round the bath tub, and as you soak let your whole body unwind.

03

8 Remember, a little exercise is better than none When you can't do all three toning exercises for a week of the programme, just do one, and congratulate yourself for managing to do something, no matter how rushed or tired you're feeling. Trea, one of our case studies, suggested fitting in a toning exercise while you're waiting for the kettle to boil – try it.

9 Manage your time Recently, a top business person gave me the following tip and it's proved invaluable: at the start of the day, do the one task you really don't want to do. Make it the first thing you do after breakfast or when you've arrived at work. When that's out of the way, you'll feel virtuous, worry-free – and will have more time for the tasks you enjoy – including exercise.

10 Enter a charity race Do this with a friend or work colleague – raise money for charity and get a great feeling of achievement. Entering a race will give you a fitness goal to work towards – if you're a beginner, your power walks will help to prepare you for the event.

BODY SCRUB

Use this body scrub recipe as a weekly treat – it's also great for exfoliating before applying fake tan.

- Half a cup of brown sugar
- The juice of half a freshly squeezed orange
- 1 tablespoon vitamin E oil

Mix the ingredients in a bowl, then take a handful and scrub into the skin all over the body in an upwards motion. Rinse off and apply moisturiser.

---

record your progress

Fill in the blanks below to chart your success.

Measurements before the start of Week 03:	Measurements at the end of Week 03:
bust	bust
waist	waist
hips	hips
thighs	thighs
upper arms	upper arms

How many power walks did you do?

1   2   3   4

How many pedometer steps?

How many toning sessions did you do?

1   2   3   4

Rate your healthy eating this week

1   2   3   4   5   (1, poor and 5, excellent)

Rate your water intake this week

1   2   3   4   5   (1, poor and 5, excellent)

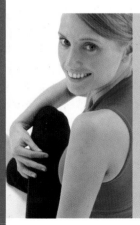

'You are halfway there now, so tighten your belt as your clothes get looser and your body is gradually becoming more toned.'

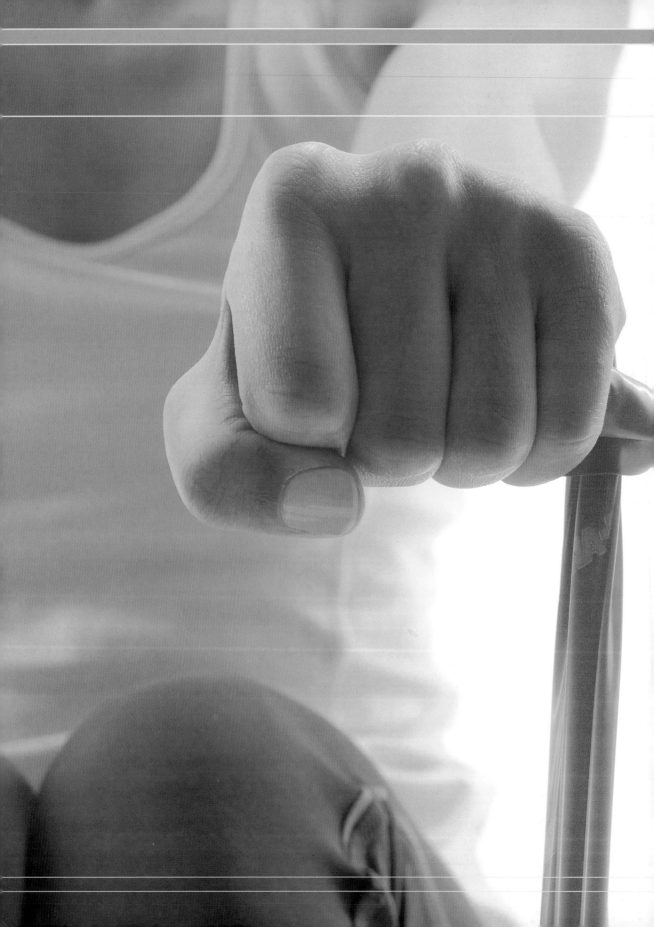

04

week 04

seated row
seated twist
squat and lift

Not only are you now looking good and feeling fantastic, but your fitness levels are improving and you will be power walking at a faster pace. Time your power walk and see how much more quickly you can cover the same distance as you did in Week 01. You can also check your pedometer steps and compare them with your total from three weeks ago.

seated row
week 04 • upper body

This is the No-Gym equivalent of the rowing machine, using two small water bottles for resistance. By holding in your abdominal muscles as you row, you build core stability while working out your arms. You'll get definition where it counts, sculpting the triceps, deltoids and biceps, and strengthening the muscles of the back.

WHAT DOES IT DO?

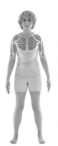

Tones the principal arm muscles – the deltoids, triceps and biceps. Tones the rhomboid and latissimus dorsi muscles of the upper, middle and lower back respectively.

calories burned	3
weekly calories	9

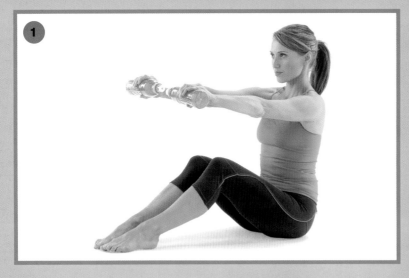

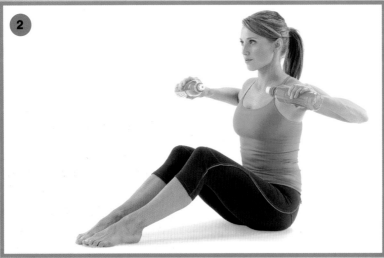

the exercise

1 Hold a water bottle in each hand. Sit with your knees up and arms extended, shoulder-width apart. Keep your shoulders down and look straight ahead.

2 Breathe in and then exhale, pushing your arms forwards and pulling back, making a rowing action. Keep your stomach muscles pulled in to support your posture and protect your back.

repeat 12–20x

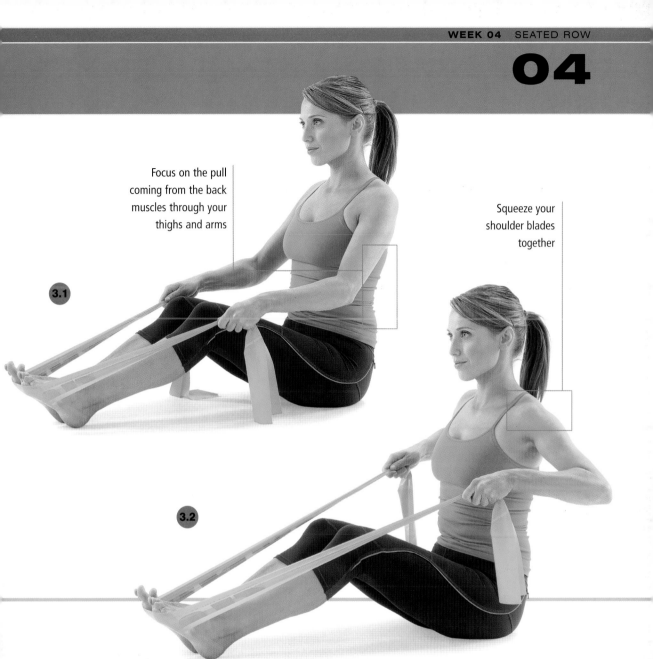

Focus on the pull coming from the back muscles through your thighs and arms

Squeeze your shoulder blades together

3.1

3.2

boost the burn

3 Hold a resistance band around your feet to increase the intensity.

repeat 12–20x

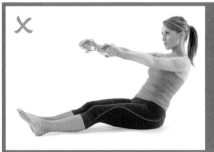

what to avoid

Don't relax the position by leaning back as then you won't benefit from the intense abdominal workout you get by adopting the correct pose.

seated twist
week 04 • middle body

The seated twist encourages good posture, draws in the waist and strengthens the deepest abdominal muscles like a corset for that hourglass figure. You'll find this move also tones the muscles that support the lower back – a tonic if you've spent too many sedentary hours at your desk.

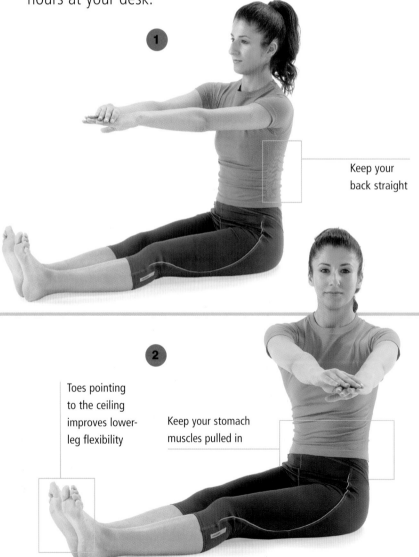

Keep your
back straight

Toes pointing
to the ceiling
improves lower-
leg flexibility

Keep your stomach
muscles pulled in

WHAT DOES IT DO?

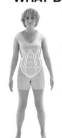

Works three major muscle groups, toning the obliques and transverse abdominis (the stomach and waist muscles) and stretching the hamstrings.

calories burned	4
weekly calories	12

the exercise

1 Sit on the floor with your legs and arms extended before you as shown, with one hand holding the opposite wrist. Sit with your back straight but relaxed and your feet flexed. Pull your navel in towards your spine. Look towards your fingertips.

2 Slowly twist to the side, hold for a count of five, then return to the starting position. Now twist to the opposite side. Repeat, alternating from side to side, doing a total of 20 twists – 10 on each side. Keep the movement slow and controlled.

repeat 12–20x

04

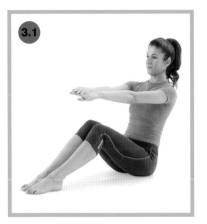

3.1

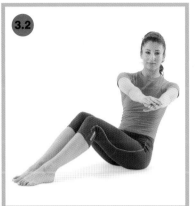

3.2

boost the burn

3 Bending your knees slightly and leaning back increases the intensity of this exercise, engaging the core transverse abdominal muscles to give a more advanced workout.

repeat 12–20x

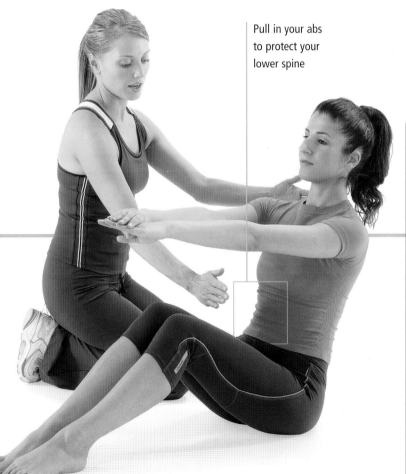

Pull in your abs to protect your lower spine

what to avoid

Don't let your back slump or twist from the hip – if you're tired, take a break and go for five twists each side rather than aim too high and let your good technique slip away. To get results, always twist from the waist, engaging the abdominal muscles, keeping your back straight.

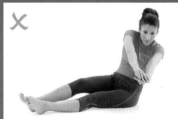

squat and lift
week 04 • lower body

The squat and lift is the perfect antidote to square-hip syndrome. Effective for defining the outer curve of the hips and bottom, this exercise works the outer hip muscle, legs and abdominals. It's a really effective way of tightening the buttocks, so if you're a pear shape make sure you add the squat and lift to your maintenance programme (see pages 134–5).

WHAT DOES IT DO?

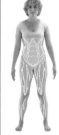

Tones the gluteus maximus muscles of the hip/buttocks, the abductor, hamstrings and quadriceps of the thighs, and the transverse abdominis muscles of the stomach.

calories burned	11
weekly calories	33

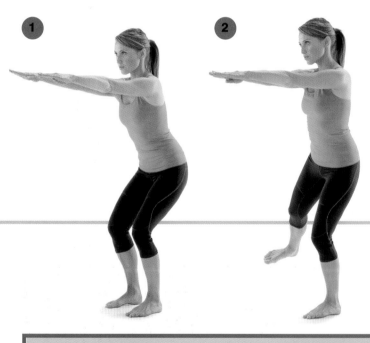

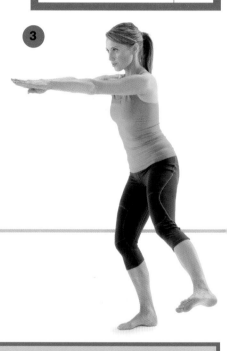

the exercise

1 Stand with your feet hip-width apart and your arms extended. Feel your weight through your heels. Breathe in, then exhale and bend as if you are about to sit on a chair, then straighten.

2 Lift one leg to the side – keep the movement controlled, and don't lift the leg too high.

3 Lower the leg then repeat the squat and lift the opposite leg. Work towards one smooth movement – squat, come up and lift.

repeat 12–20x

04

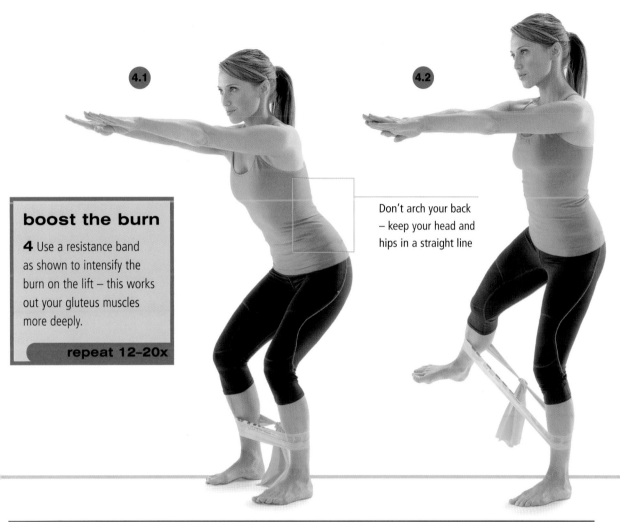

4.1

4.2

boost the burn

4 Use a resistance band as shown to intensify the burn on the lift – this works out your gluteus muscles more deeply.

repeat 12–20x

Don't arch your back – keep your head and hips in a straight line

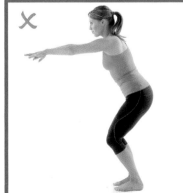

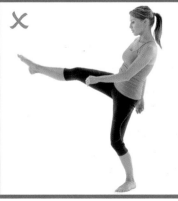

what to avoid

Don't lock out your knees or let your knees extend beyond your toes.

Don't kick above the level of your waist.

case study • Karen

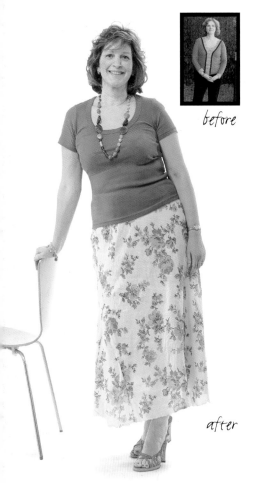

before

after

Name: Karen
Age: 49
Lifestyle: Living with husband. Working full time as a dental hygienist. Three children, aged 14, 19 and 27.

'Two years ago, my daughter got married and I lost weight for the wedding,' Karen began. 'But since then the weight has piled back on.' She began the six-week plan because, like many people, she felt that she had to do something, particularly about her expanding upper arms and waist. But she certainly didn't expect to enjoy it. 'At first,' she confided, 'I just thought, "Let's get it over with," but after a couple of weeks I started to accept the exercises as a part of my working life. And I found them easy to fit around my routine.'

It was the power walking that took Karen most by surprise. 'I've never been sporty and, I'm ashamed to say, I've never done any real exercise before. But I loved the power walks, and I'm going to keep doing them even when I'm happy with my weight.' Karen found she could fit them in at lunchtime, and was able to keep walking at a brisk pace because her time was limited.

A new goal that's fuelling Karen's motivation is her 30th wedding anniversary. She will be celebrating with her husband in India, and this trip has become a real incentive to keep exercising, as well as to cut down on the rich food she loves. 'I eat fruit instead of puddings and limit carbs in the evenings, as I find this really works for me,' she says.

Since following the programme, Karen has lost weight, toned up (although she decided not to measure herself) and has more energy in the

'I loved the power walks, and I'm going to keep doing them even when I'm happy with my weight'

mornings. 'Lucy's programme has also really helped me with hot flushes – as I'm getting fitter, they seem to be happening less often,' she says.

Karen believes that Lucy's reassurance that she could miss some of the programme and still succeed helped her to keep going. 'Around week three I was ill for a few days. Lucy told me to leave the exercising until I felt completely better. I still lost weight and what was interesting was that I missed the power walking, and really wanted to get back to it.'

the results

No measurements taken; preferred the scales.

Starting weight: **75.5kg (12st)**
After six weeks: **71.5kg (11st 5lb)**
Loss: **4.1kg (9lb)**

questions and answers

How do I get rid of my bingo wings?

Bingo wings – the flabby area at the backs of your upper arms – are very common, but they're not difficult areas to tone when you know what to do. First, use hand weights while you're power walking. Secondly, the box press (see page 48) and the overhead arm press (see page 72) are great for toning the backs of the arms. And thirdly, you could do two upper body exercises each week rather than one.

Will exercise increase my appetite?

This is a common myth, but the answer is no, not at all! What you will find is that you will probably drink a lot more water (which helps to eliminate toxins from your body and improves your skin – see page 23). Regular exercise can help to control your appetite – and the better you feel, the better your diet.

I want to tone my inner thighs – should I measure my thighs each week?

The No-Gym Workout will help you to get slender thighs. To keep things simple, I recommend measuring the upper, middle and lower body (which also relates to the exercises, which generally fall into upper, middle and lower-body categories). However, if measuring your thighs will motivate you, just measure the widest part of one thigh, and measure at the same place each week. If you have an obvious freckle or mark, use this as a reminder of where to measure.

With every diet I go on, my weight fluctuates. Why is this diet different?

The good news is that this programme is not a diet, but a way of life that fits in with you. It's safe with realistic goals, and you'll be able to manage your weight more effectively because you'll be eating sensibly and exercising to increase your metabolic rate. Fad diets often mean losing muscle instead of fat, which slow down your metabolic rate and inhibit weight loss.

At what stage should I undertake the 'boost the burn' exercises?

If you can do 20 repetitions of an exercise with complete ease, move on to boost the burn. You can also test your effort level to see if you're ready to work harder: if your effort level is 4 or less, it's time to rev up (see the intensity chart on page 43). Generally, you should be working at effort level 5 to 6, so if this applies to you, don't move on to boost the burn – you're getting enough of a workout doing the standard exercises.

Another way to up the intensity – and this applies to any exercise within the programme – is to keep your movements slow and controlled, with your abdominal muscles pulled in tight. Pulling your abs tight to your spine when you're doing upper-body toning, for example, gives you a faster, more effective workout. You're effectively doing two exercises in one, which saves you valuable time.

I find it hard to motivate myself to exercise after a day's work. How can I stay focused?

If you are tired and stressed when you walk in the door from work, then this is the best time to exercise away your stress and boost your energy levels. Motivate yourself by putting on your favourite upbeat CD and use some of the visualisation techniques on pages 80–1. I promise that you will feel great during and after exercise – and so much better than if you had crashed on the sofa, which simply leads to an energy decline. When you expend energy, you generate energy, and this in turn will make your evening more enjoyable.

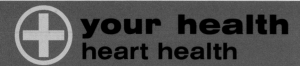

your health
heart health

Your heart is the core of your physical being, and in modern Western culture, a gauge of emotional health that is a symbol of our feelings, from heartbroken to heartless, heartened to heartfelt. In Britain, around 140,000 people die every year of heart disease. Yet with lifestyle changes such as regular exercise and improved diet, you can greatly reduce your potential for heart problems.

More men suffer from heart problems when young, but after menopause women are at increased risk of experiencing heart conditions. As with many serious conditions, such as osteoporosis (see pages 68–9), take action when you're younger and you decrease your risk.

Begin, or continue, with exercise and a good diet throughout your life and you'll be giving yourself the best possible chance of avoiding debilitating and potentially life-threatening disease. If you have a predisposition towards certain conditions, such as heart disease, it's all the more reason to protect your body for the future. If you have had heart problems, however, don't undertake any exercise programme without first consulting your doctor.

**THE BENEFITS OF
REGULAR EXERCISE**

- Fights high LDL cholesterol levels

- Improves circulation

- Lowers blood pressure

- Helps to protect against heart disease and other serious conditions, such as breast cancer

- Extends your life expectancy by an average of seven years

---

why your 20-minute power walk is a heart-saver

A growing body of scientific research has shown that regular exercise can reduce the risk of heart problems by 30–50 per cent. In a study of more than 70,000 women published in the *New England Journal of Medicine*, those who walked for a minimum of 2½ hours a week (around 20 minutes a day) reduced their likelihood of heart problems by 30 per cent. If the women walked more than this they further reduced their risk of heart problems and other serious conditions, but just 20 minutes a day was all it took to make a real difference.

balancing cholesterol

The majority of people who have heart disease suffer from high cholesterol. There are three types of cholesterol, or fats, in the blood: LDL (low density lipoprotein), HDL (high density lipoprotein) and triglycerides or VLDL (very low density lipoprotein). LDL and VLDL are looked upon as the 'bad' lipids, in that they are deposited into artery walls. HDL is the 'good' lipid, as it is the mechanism by which fats are carried away from the bloodstream to be excreted by the liver. We usually have more LDL and VLDL than HDL and the ratio between them matters. The crucial measurement is the ratio of total cholesterol (the sum of the HDL, LDL and VLDL) to HDL. If the total cholesterol count is five times or more higher than the HDL level, then it is too high, and needs to be lowered. The aim is to try to bring it to 3:1. At 5:1 or more, the total cholesterol to HDL ratio is too high

KEEP YOUR HEART IN SHAPE

To keep your heart healthy you don't need to spend hours at the gym – simply make these small but significant changes to your routine and your heart will love you for it. Remember, always check with your doctor before taking exercise if you have ever experienced heart problems or are at potential risk.

• Power walk halfway to work three times a week – use public transport to get you the rest of the way or back home.

• If you work in an office, use the stairs not the lift. Count the stairs you climb and add them to your weekly checkouts along with your pedometer steps.

• Walk briskly and monitor your effort level – see the Borg scale on page 43.

and the excess LDL cholesterol in the arteries is deposited in their walls. This narrows them, increasing the risk of heart disease and stroke. Aerobic exercise decreases LDL cholesterol and triglycerides and raises HDL, as does eating fewer saturated fats, which include butter and red meats.

improving circulation

Exercise increases your heart rate, so your heart pumps more blood around your body. This helps to keep your arteries clear of blood clots and discourages the build up of fat, which can cause the narrowing of blood vessels linked with conditions such as angina.

lowering blood pressure

High blood pressure, or hypertension, is linked with heart disease and stroke. Regular exercise and a diet low in saturated fat and caffeine help to reduce hypertension.

record your progress

Fill in the blanks below to chart your success.

Measurements before the start of Week 04:	Measurements at the end of Week 04:
bust	bust
waist	waist
hips	hips
thighs	thighs
upper arms	upper arms

How many power walks did you do?

1   2   3   4

How many pedometer steps?

How many toning sessions did you do?

1   2   3   4

Rate your healthy eating this week

1   2   3   4   5   (1, poor and 5, excellent)

Rate your water intake this week

1   2   3   4   5   (1, poor and 5, excellent)

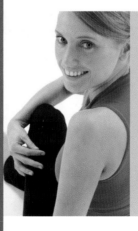

'You have made exercise part of your life. How fantastic does it feel to know that you will now always feel toned and energised?'

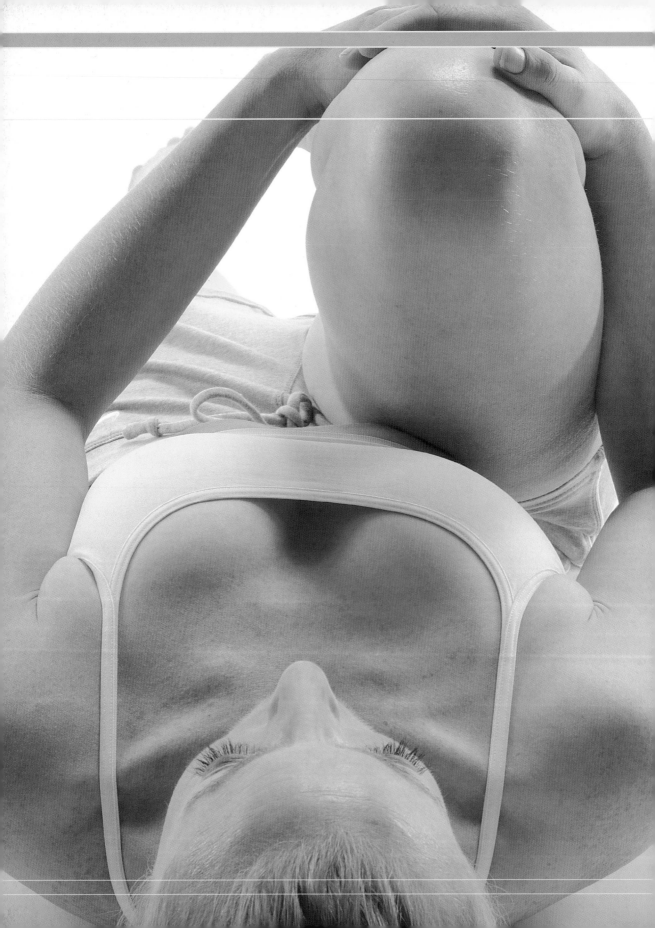

05

week 05

criss-cross arms
abdominal roll
gluteal circle

You are now a regular exerciser and you are turning back the years in how you look and feel every time you exercise. Feel proud of yourself and your achievements so far, and make sure you keep your focus as you work through the last two weeks of the programme.

criss-cross arms
week 05 • upper body

This arm exercise firms the muscles of the chest, toning the supporting muscles around the bust. Also a remedy for squidgy upper arms, you'll feel the stretch all the way from your shoulders to your fingertips as sleeping muscles stir into action. Make sure you keep your abdominal muscles pulled in for maximum benefit to your stomach, back and posture.

WHAT DOES IT DO?

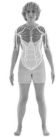

Tones the biceps and triceps of the arms, the pectoralis major muscle of the chest and the transversus abdominis muscle of the stomach.

calories burned	5
weekly calories	15

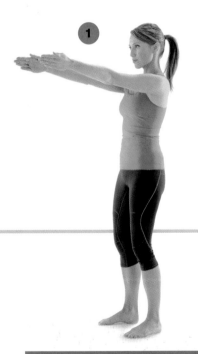

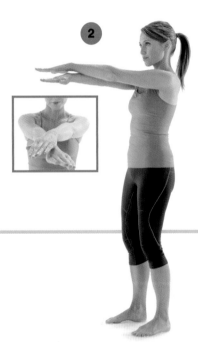

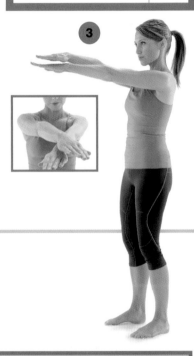

the exercise

1 Stand with your arms extended in front of you, your palms facing each other.

2 Breathe in then exhale as you cross your left arm over your right arm, turning your palms down along the way. Pause for a moment, then return to the starting position and repeat.

3 Repeat the set on the other side, this time crossing your right arm over your left.

repeat 12–20x

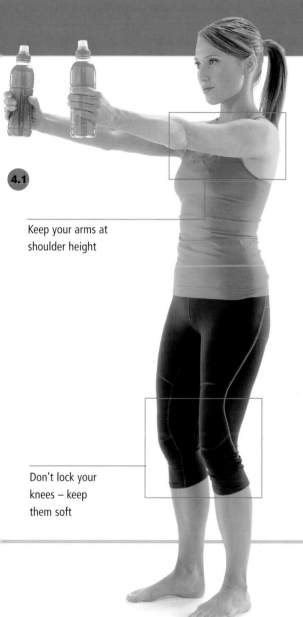

4.1

Keep your arms at
shoulder height

Don't lock your
knees – keep
them soft

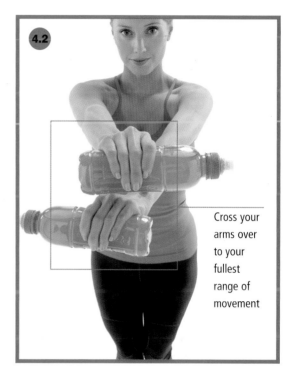

4.2

Cross your
arms over
to your
fullest
range of
movement

boost the burn

4 Do the basic exercise but
use filled water bottles or hand
weights to increase the intensity
in the upper arms.

repeat 12–20x

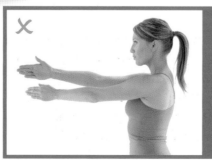

what to avoid

Don't have your palms facing
inwards and up – they need to be
horizontal. Keep your arms straight.
Use your abdominal muscles to
maintain good posture.

abdominal roll
week 05 • middle body

The ab roll works every part of every abdominal muscle you possess – provided you develop a good, precise technique. The key to an intense abdominal workout is using your breath to power each movement, breathing out on the 'effort', when you roll your upper body towards your knees, and breathing in on the release.

WHAT DOES IT DO?

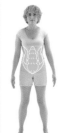

Works the rectus abdominis and transversus abdominis muscles of the stomach and the obliques of the waist.

calories burned	2
weekly calories	6

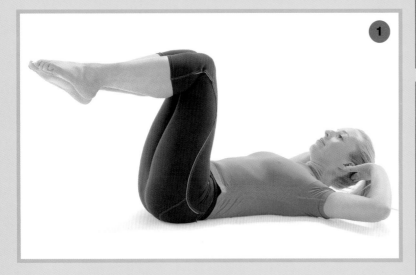

1

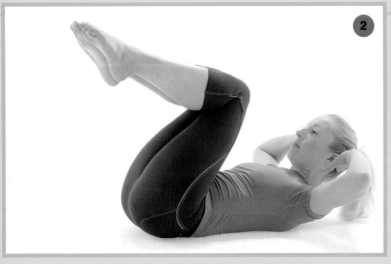

2

the exercise

1 Lie on the floor, with knees raised and feet together. Keep your knees level with your hips, forming a right angle. Breathe in.

2 With fingertips touching your ears and your elbows out, breathe out as you raise your head, shoulders and upper back towards your knees. Pull in the abdominal muscles, imagining your navel touching your spine.

variation

If you suffer from back or neck problems, cross your arms behind your head with your hands on the tops of your shoulders and arms snug under your neck for support (see page 50).

repeat 12–20x

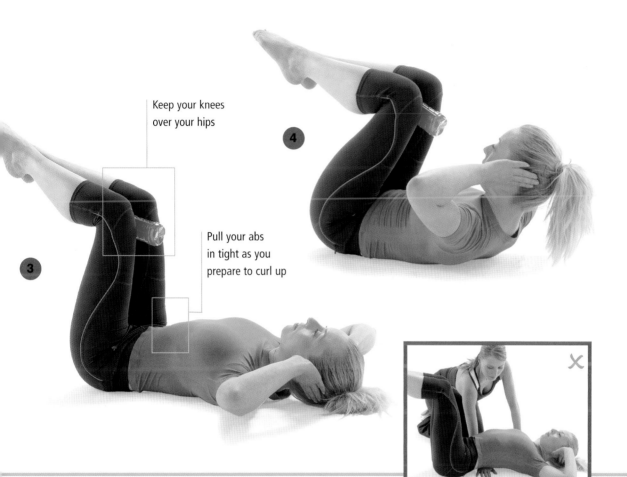

Keep your knees
over your hips

4

Pull your abs
in tight as you
prepare to curl up

3

what to avoid

Always make sure that your lower
back is touching the floor. Check
by pausing to see if you can slide a
hand under this part of your back,
or ask a friend to do this for you.
Begin the exercise again, this time
working slowly so your lower back
has complete floor contact.

boost the burn

3 Use a hand weight or bottle of water, gripping it between your upper
knees. Raise your body towards your knees, but do it super slow – lift
and lower for a count of four.

4 For even more intensity, start the ab roll a few inches from the floor and
slowly raise your body towards your knees.

repeat 12–20x

gluteal circle
week 05 • lower body

The gluteal circle, practised by dancers, improves posture and intensely works the thighs, buttocks and abdominals. The rotation improves hip mobility and tones the hip area. Soon you won't need tight jeans to contain cellulite-stricken thighs and bottom, as the gluteal circle also firms and lifts the buttocks. This elegant exercise can also work your abdominals by keeping them pulled in as you extend your leg behind, to the side and in front.

WHAT DOES IT DO?

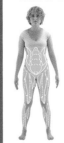

Tones the gluteal muscles of the hips/buttocks, tones quadriceps, hamstrings and abductors of the working leg, the abs, and the muscles of the standing leg.

calories burned	12
weekly calories	36

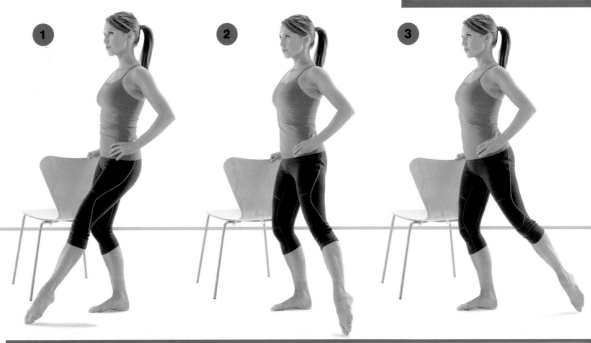

the exercise

1 Standing on your right leg, extend your left leg in front of you, using a chair to help maintain your balance. Breathe evenly throughout the exercise.

2 Squeeze your left gluteals (hip/buttock muscles) and slowly sweep your left leg to the side, keeping the abdominal muscles pulled in.

3 Maintaining the squeeze, circle your left leg behind.

repeat 12–20x

05

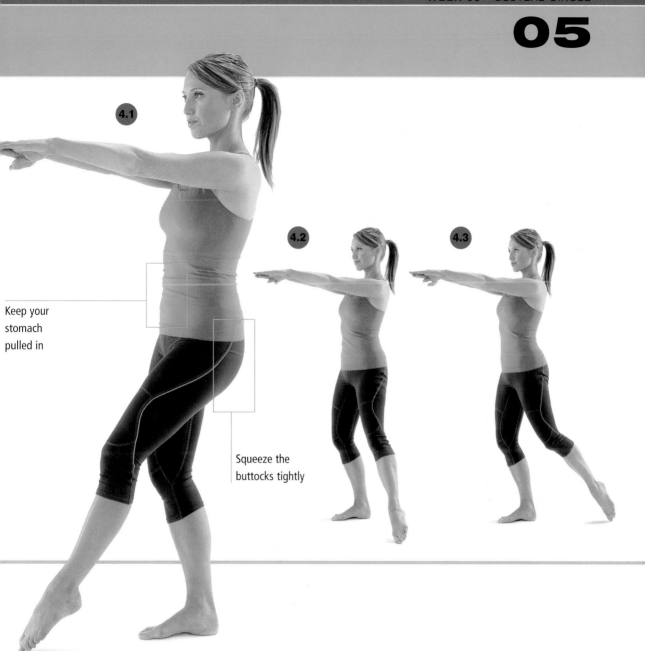

4.1

Keep your
stomach
pulled in

Squeeze the
buttocks tightly

4.2

4.3

boost the burn

4 Perform the exercise without a chair – this gets the stomach and thigh muscles of the moving leg working more intensely. Also, increase your range of movement, making a wider arc. You could use water bottles as markers to give you points to aim for as you circle your leg.

repeat 12–20x

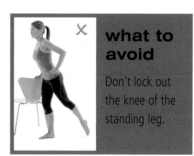

X

what to avoid

Don't lock out the knee of the standing leg.

case study · Jess

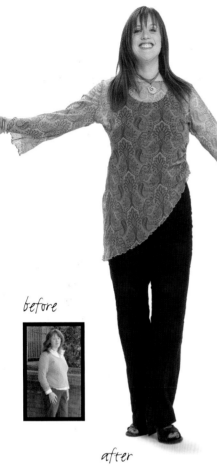

before

after

Name: Jess

Age: 33

Lifestyle: Living with husband. Mother of three children, aged six-and-a-half, five, and 11 months. Recently started up her own business.

'Exercise videos or DVDs just don't work, not when you have kids,' Jess began, 'but with the No-Gym Workout I could do all the exercises at home and the weekly goals were achievable.'

Jess's weight concerns began after having children – she really wanted to flatten her stomach, so her health visitor recommended that she attend a local authority gym. 'I hated it,' Jess confided, 'The ethos was total vanity; lots of preening in mirrors and I didn't even make it through the induction.'

Jess began the No-Gym Workout, and quickly found she could fit in the exercises around the children. 'I also adapted the press-ups by practising them on the bed, which has less impact on my joints but still works my abs.' Jess found the power walking harder to fit in, but devised a solution by power walking on a trampette while watching television with her family.

Jess also has to spend additional time planning meals because her children have food allergies, so she is nut-free, dairy-free, wheat- and gluten-free. 'It's a tough diet to maintain at

times, but it did kickstart my weight loss,' she explains. 'I also have an under-active thyroid, so the eating regime at home plus the No-Gym Workout will help me in the long term, keeping my metabolism more active.' Even while taking thyroxin, Jess's metabolism can drop as low as 40 per cent below normal.

Measuring was off the agenda for Jess. 'I've always been a bit neurotic about the scales,' Jess says, 'in fact, my husband wanted to take them off me at one stage because I was using

'I adapted the press-ups by practising them on the bed, which has less impact on my joints but still works my abs'

them all the time.' Jess limited herself to stepping on the scales once a week during the six weeks, but chose not to take her measurements.

'I'm delighted with the results,' Jess smiles. 'Already, I feel better – and I'm back to the weight I was before having my third baby, Amelia.'

the results

No measurements taken; preferred the scales.

Starting weight: **83kg (13st 2lb)**

After six weeks: **75.5kg (12st)**

Loss: **7.5kg (1st 2lb)**

questions and answers

I want to tone and strengthen my legs. How can I achieve quicker results while power walking?

Power walking is a great way to tone your legs, but I strongly advise you not to walk with ankle weights, as they can cause injury to the lower body. The way to increase resistance while power walking is by using hand weights (see pages 30 and 36). If you complete your three walks a week and do your toning exercises, you will see results quickly anyway. You could also add an extra lower body exercise to your circuit if you prefer.

Can exercise help me to reduce the feeling of stress in my life?

Totally. One of the best benefits of regular exercise is stress reduction and mood enhancement. Exercise not only makes you look good, but it makes you feel good, too.

Is it true that muscle weighs more than fat?

It's true – muscle is more dense than fat, so it weighs more than the same volume of fat. Two people can be the same height and share the same physical measurements, but the person who has more fat will actually weigh less. This is why I recommend measuring as a way to monitor your progress, as opposed to weighing yourself on the scales.

What is core strength?

Core strength refers to the strength of your torso – the centre of your body, including the abdominal muscles, obliques and lower back. Core strength is important for general health and fitness and makes you less prone to injury. This is why throughout the book there is a constant reminder to engage your core muscles by pulling your belly button in tight to your spine. Without a strong core, your fitness potential is limited – you will only be able to improve your fitness to a certain point.

I have a three-month-old baby. When can I move from the postnatal programme to the full workout?

I would recommend that you check with your doctor before you progress to the next stage, then start with the easier versions of the workout. Pay extra attention to keeping your abdominal muscles pulled in tight to help strengthen the stomach muscles.

Can I buy resistance bands on the high street?

Most good high-street sports stores stock resistance bands. You can also find them on the internet just by typing in the name. They vary in resistance, from beginners to advanced. I recommend you go for beginners or intermediate.

I can't leave my children at home so it's difficult to find the time to power walk. Can they come too?

Absolutely – get the whole family fit and you will all benefit. You could play games while power walking with your children. For example, walk in single file then everyone has to walk fast and whoever is at the back has to overtake and get to the front. You can also get them to play I-spy or sing a song. Using a bit of imagination will make it an adventure for them and a calorie burn for you.

Will toning training help to improve my posture?

Toning does help to improve your posture. It strengthens your skeletal muscles and makes your bones stronger. This strength helps your body to sit and stand.

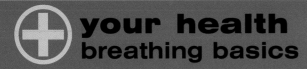

your health
breathing basics

We breathe more than 350 million times over an average lifespan, feeding ourselves with oxygen and expelling carbon dioxide, yet we pay little attention to the quiet rise and fall of our breathing throughout our lives. In Sanskrit, the ancient language of the yoga sutras, breath or prana means respiration, and also life, energy or strength. It describes how breathing techniques can be an amazing way to energise your body, achieve relaxation and focus your mind.

breathing through the burn

When you exercise, you need to breathe more deeply, and sometimes more rapidly, than usual to give your body the oxygen it needs to provide the required energy for your level of physical activity. In many exercises you breathe out on the 'effort', when you feel that burn or resistance in your muscles. Check that you're breathing at the right stage of the exercise, and that you're breathing correctly – taking deep breaths in through your nose and exhaling through your mouth – as doing so will make the effort feel easier.

Breath control also helps you to feel in control of your body. There's a tendency nowadays to 'just do it' – literally – which some people interpret as holding their breath until the exercise is over, without really thinking about what they are doing or enjoying the process of exercising. I advise my clients to use their awareness of their breathing as a way of getting in touch with how they are feeling during exercise. Being more sensitive to your body in this way will help you to make better judgments about how many repetitions of an exercise you can do, and when you need to stop.

ENERGISING BREATH TECHNIQUE

Deep breathing both relaxes and energises your body. Whenever you're tired during your workout, stop, take a drink of water and practise this energising breathing technique. It takes less than a minute, and you can practise it anywhere at any time. It also works whenever you're feeling an energy low – try it while sitting at your desk mid-afternoon, while you're standing in a queue, or simply for motivation when you've got a million things to do but just can't get started.

1. Lie on your back. Close your eyes and place your palms face downwards on the floor. Let your spine sink into the floor.

2. Relax the muscles of your face and jaw by letting your mouth fall open.

3. Take a long, deep breath. Breathe in deeply and slowly through your nose, filling the bottom of your lungs; avoid shallow-breathing only into your chest. Feel your lungs expand in all directions. Exhale slowly through your mouth, imagining a column of air rising through you.

4. Repeat four times, so you have taken a total of five deep breaths.

5. Now open your eyes and stand up slowly. Shake out your arms and legs to wake up your body, and you're ready to resume your workout or continue your day.

05

walking and breathing

Walking in the fresh air gives your body an oxygen boost and wakes up your circulation – there's nothing like the reconstituted air of an office to make you feel lethargic. Take deep breaths as you walk – if you begin to feel tired, count the length of your natural breaths. For example, as you inhale you might count 1, 2, 3, and again up to three when you exhale, with a count of 1 or 2 as you're about to inhale again. Now repeat and see if you can inhale and count to 4, this time inhaling more deeply and exhaling more slowly. It's a good way to train yourself to breathe deeply, keeping you feeling focused and relaxed as you walk.

breathing through a stitch The cause of a stitch is not fully known, but may be due to the pull of your internal organs on your diaphragm, induced by motion. Build your walking pace steadily and if you get a stitch, slow down or stop, bend forward and take deep breaths. Rest or continue at a slower pace until it has gone.

ANXIETY-BEATING BREATH-AWARENESS TECHNIQUE

This breath-awareness technique, the lynchpin of many types of yoga and meditation, can help you to de-stress, because you switch your focus from the worry to your physical breathing, moving your mind from your thoughts into your body. This takes practice, but it is well worth the effort.

1. Follow steps 1 and 2 opposite. Take long, deep breaths, in through your nose and out through your mouth. Every time a thought or worry intrudes, shift your focus back to your breathing.

2. Continue for as long as you need to.

---

record your progress

Fill in the blanks below to chart your success.

Measurements before the start of Week 05:	Measurements at the end of Week 05:
bust	bust
waist	waist
hips	hips
thighs	thighs
upper arms	upper arms

How many power walks did you do?

1   2   3   4

How many pedometer steps?

How many toning sessions did you do?

1   2   3   4

Rate your healthy eating this week

1   2   3   4   5   (1, poor and 5, excellent)

Rate your water intake this week

1   2   3   4   5   (1, poor and 5, excellent)

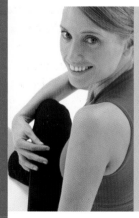

'Not only will you be looking good now and feeling full of life, but you will have improved the health of your heart and lungs so keep going!'

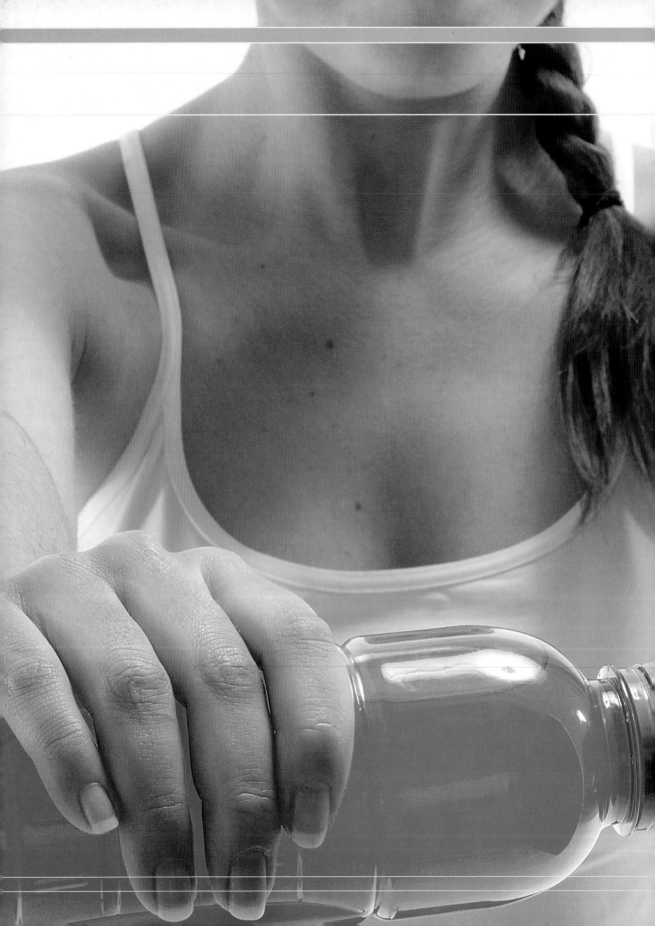

06

week 06

lateral raise
the plank
the bridge

You have reached week 06 of the programme and will now be feeling as well as seeing the results of all your hard work. Your energy levels will be raised and your increased fitness means you will be finding the exercises easier – don't forget to boost the burn when you can.

lateral raise
week 06 • upper body

This is the ultimate upper-arm exercise, working the triceps deeply. The movement is tiny but intense – you may want to begin with water bottles one-third full, then once you can do 20 reps, increase the water levels to half full and beyond. Keep your lower body relaxed.

WHAT DOES IT DO?

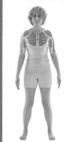

Works the triceps and deltoid muscles of the arms, the latissimus dorsi muscle of the back and the abdominals.

calories burned	5
weekly calories	15

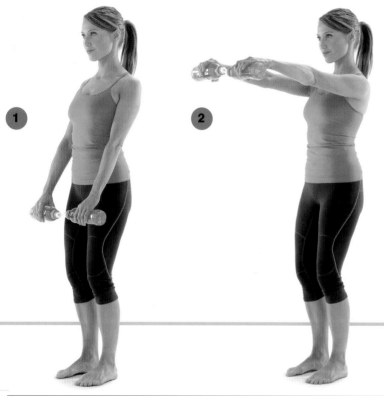

the exercise

1 Stand with your knees soft and your arms loosely by your sides. Holding a water bottle in each hand, turn your hands to the front so your palms face the front of your thighs. Pull in your abdominal muscles.

2 Breathe in and as you breathe out slowly lift your arms up to shoulder height. Hold for a couple of seconds, then in a controlled manner slowly lower your arms back to the start position. Engage the abs as you lift your arms to protect your back from pressure.

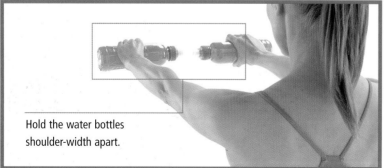

Hold the water bottles shoulder-width apart.

repeat 12–20x

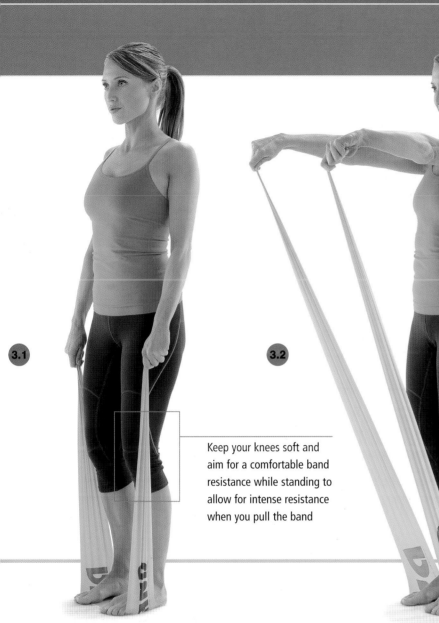

3.1

3.2

As you pull up, you work through the triceps and shoulders

Keep your knees soft and aim for a comfortable band resistance while standing to allow for intense resistance when you pull the band

boost the burn

3 Use a resistance band to increase the intensity. Stand on the band, gripping each end as you pull upwards. Keep your abdominal muscles pulled in.

repeat 12–20x

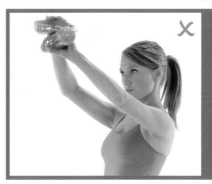

what to avoid

Don't raise your arms too high or arch your back — keep your stomach pulled in. Make sure you don't turn your hands inwards or let your arms drift.

the plank
week 06 • middle body

This is an advanced exercise, hence it is the final middle-body exercise in the No-Gym Workout. It strengthens the lower back and the 'corset' muscles, but you'll need reasonably toned abdominal muscles to begin with to be able to hold the position. The plank is renowned for improving muscular endurance, aligning the body and supporting good posture.

WHAT DOES IT DO?

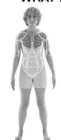

Tones the shoulder muscles, arm muscles and the deepest abdominal muscles.

calories burned	2
weekly calories	6

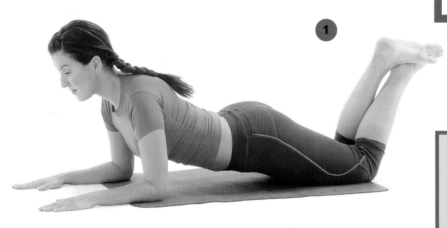

the exercise

1 Position yourself so only your hands, elbows and knees are in contact with the floor. Cross your feet. Look straight ahead and slightly down, so you don't strain your neck.

2 Pull in your abdominal muscles. Focus on creating a straight line from your shoulders to your knees. Keep your stomach muscles taut to maintain the position, pulling your navel tight to your spine. Hold for 5–10 seconds.

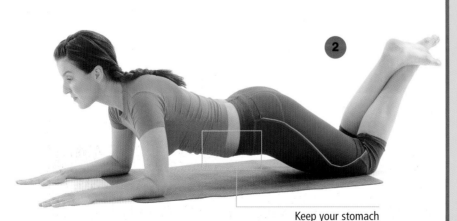

Keep your stomach muscles taut

repeat 12–20x

06

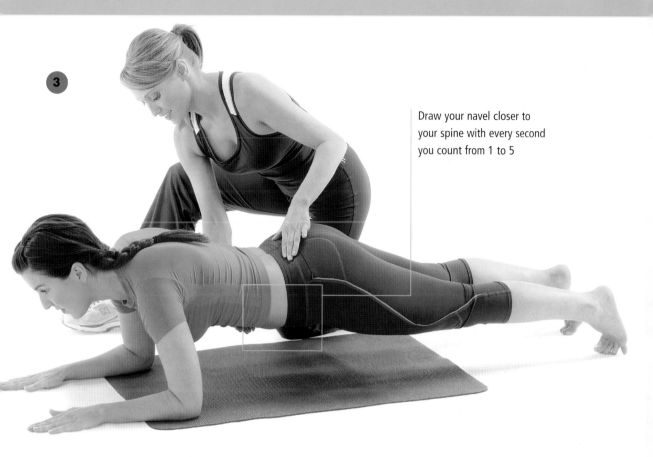

3

Draw your navel closer to your spine with every second you count from 1 to 5

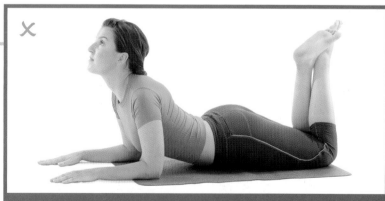

boost the burn

3 Get into the basic position, resting on your knees and elbows. Now push up onto your toes, again using your abdominal muscles to protect your back as you hold the position for 5–10 seconds. This exercise is very advanced – if you feel any discomfort or pain, stop immediately and rest; don't continue with the exercise.

repeat 12–20x

what to avoid

Don't arch your back. Don't lift your head up as this puts pressure on your back. Keep your abdominal muscles pulled in to protect your back.

the bridge
week 06 • lower body

One in three women suffers from weak pelvic floor muscles. The bridge helps to tone the pelvic floor and stomach, because by holding the position you need to engage the sling of muscles that comprises the pelvic floor, along with all the abdominals. It's also great for relieving tension in the lower back, and giving you a wobble-free, firm bottom.

WHAT DOES IT DO?

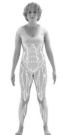

Tones the gluteus maximus on the hips/buttocks, the hamstrings and the transversus abdominis of the stomach.

calories burned	4
weekly calories	12

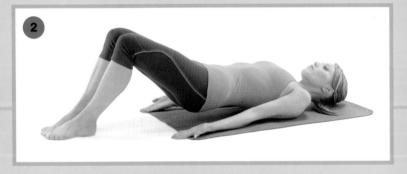

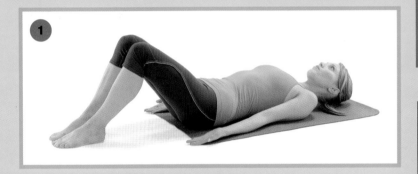

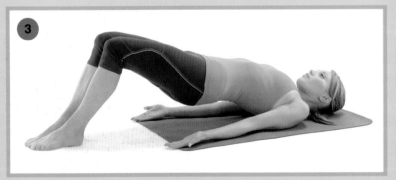

the exercise

1 Lie on your back, knees bent and feet flat on the floor, arms by your side palms facing up. Breathe in.

2 Exhale as you contract your buttock muscles and press your weight through your heels. Slowly raise your hips off the floor. Keep your navel pulled in to your spine to prevent your lower back from dipping.

3 Keep lifting, so you fully extend your body from your knees through your upper body. Pull in your abdominal and buttock muscles, squeeze your thighs and hold the position for 2–3 seconds, then release.

repeat 12–20x

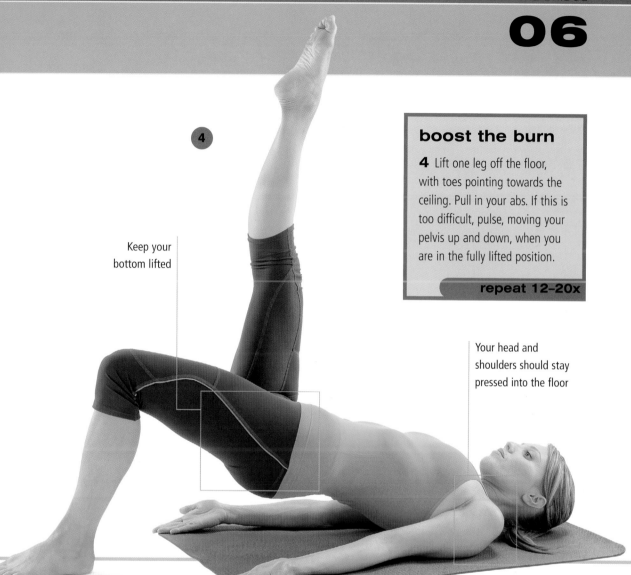

4

Keep your
bottom lifted

boost the burn

4 Lift one leg off the floor, with toes pointing towards the ceiling. Pull in your abs. If this is too difficult, pulse, moving your pelvis up and down, when you are in the fully lifted position.

repeat 12–20x

Your head and
shoulders should stay
pressed into the floor

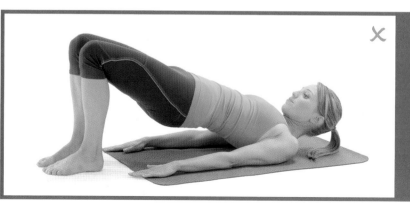

✕

what to avoid

Don't lift your head off the floor. Also, keep your back in a straight line. Here, the knees are too far out and the feet are pointing inwards. Don't let your feet stray too far from your body, and have your palms facing up, not down.

case study · Trea

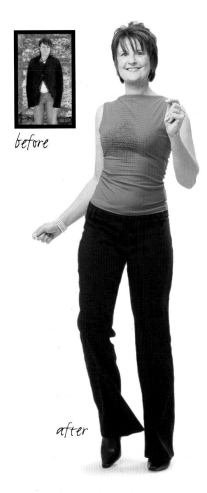

before

after

Name: Trea
Age: 39
Lifestyle: Living with partner. Works full-time as a teaching assistant. Two grown-up children.

'I used to be a size 10, but over the last three years I've grown to be a borderline size 14,' Trea begins. 'I work in a school and school dinners have been my downfall – I have been eating two main meals a day!'

As a teaching assistant Trea has an active role in the classroom, but she drives to work and was taking virtually no exercise. 'I got lazy, I suppose, because when I was younger I was eight-and-a-half stone and could eat anything, but once I got past the age of 32 something changed, and it became harder to keep weight off.

'Next year I hit 40,' she continues, 'and I decided that was as good a reason as any to tone up and get back to my old shape.' There was also a health reason for starting the No-Gym Workout to get fit and lose weight – Trea's mother is diabetic, and other members of the family suffer from Type I and Type II diabetes.

'The exercises were so easy to fit in,' Trea explains. 'I'd do the lunge and kick in the kitchen while waiting for the kettle to boil. You can always find a gap in the day to tone, even while watching television. There just wasn't a good excuse not to.'

Trea's other tip is to break down the exercise. For example, doing the lower-body one in the morning, middle body at lunchtime and upper body before dinner. This is a great way to cover the exercises in the space of a day when you have limited time or your motivation is low.

She tackled the power walks by gathering others to walk with her during their lunch break. 'About nine of us all go out together, and it's great fun,' she says.

'The exercises were so easy to fit in. I'd do the lunge and kick in the kitchen while waiting for the kettle to boil'

Trea lost an amazing 20cm (8in) off her waist, and is now down to a comfortable size 10. She didn't make any drastic changes to her diet, other than limit her portions and increase her water intake.

What motivated Trea most was her fast progress. 'At week one I could do four press-ups, but by week six I could do 21,' she says with a smile.

the results

Centimetre/inch loss after six weeks:

Bust: **5cm (2in)**
Waist: **20cm (8in)**
Hips: **5cm (2in)**
Thighs: **2.5cm (1in)**
Upper arms: **stayed the same**

questions and answers

I am exercising regularly and finding I am getting ravenous between workouts. What is the best way to handle this?

First, as you are exercising regularly, make sure that you are drinking plenty of water, as deyhydration can sometimes be confused with hunger. The more exercise you do, the more calories you burn so you need to refuel your body. Be sure to make healthy food choices – for example, bananas and nuts are a great way to combat hunger, so keep some handy at home or in your handbag or desk drawer at work to avoid the temptation of sugar- or fat-laden nibbles (see pages 40–1 for instant healthy snacks).

How can I use a stability ball to enhance my workouts?

You can use a stability ball, or Swiss ball, to tone your abdominals while practising the upper-body exercises – simply sit on the ball with good posture as you do the arm exercises. Because your body naturally uses its core muscles (those of your waist and stomach) to stop you rolling off the ball, you'll get a great abdominal workout with simultaneous upper-body toning. Just sitting on a stability ball without doing anything else works your deepest abdominal muscles and improves your posture; some of my clients sit on one while watching television, and it really helps to tone a wobbly tummy.

Can I continue doing the No-Gym Workout while I'm on holiday?

Definitely. You can do the exercises easily in your hotel room, villa or apartment, so make a note of three or six toning exercises (depending on if you'll be away for one week or two) or colour-copy the visual index on pages 136–9. If you're staying near a beach, you could do your power walking on the sand, which is more of a challenge, and fantastic for toning the legs. For variation, swap a power walk for a good 20-minute swim.

Can my partner join me on the programme?

It's great to train with someone else, so yes, absolutely. When power walking, your partner may want to invest in hand weights so that he can get a good upper-body workout while he walks; also, he'll be able to use the hand weights for the upper-body exercises so he has more resistance to work with. You'll enjoy power walking together as you can motivate each other; and it's always safer being outdoors with a companion.

Is there an exercise I can do to lift my bust?

Yes. Although exercise cannot increase bust size, you can certainly combat gravity by practising specific exercises to tone the pectorals – the muscles principally responsible for the pertness of the breasts. The elbow and bust press (see page 60) targets these muscles to help lift and draw the breasts together. All the upper-body exercises in this book have this age-defying effect.

Is it essential to power walk three times a week on the maintenance programme?

One of the case studies, Trea, lives five minutes away from me and I still see her out power walking all the time as it is part of her life now. She has felt the benefits and says she never wants to go back to feeling lethargic and unhappy with her weight. I would recommend that you always aim for three walks a week although missing the odd one won't hurt. If you prefer, you can always replace one walk with another form of aerobic exercise such as swimming, cycling or aerobics.

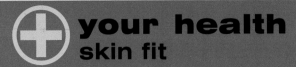

your health
skin fit

Exercise is a great way to ensure fantastic-looking skin. By exercising regularly, you'll improve your circulation, which stimulates blood flow to the skin, promoting the elimination of natural waste products, and giving you a brighter, radiant complexion. A few small changes to your daily skincare routine can also make a big difference to the long-term health of your skin. Here's how to give your skin the best possible attention.

Your skin is your barrier against the outside world, protecting you from harmful UV light, pollutants and bacteria, regulating body temperature and showing you what's happening on the inside, too, as an indicator of your general health. Adequate cover against the sun's rays, eating and drinking sensibly, not smoking and simple skincare can help you to guard against skin damage and keep your skin looking younger for longer.

protect your skin every day

While you're out power walking, you'll need to use a SPF sunscreen to protect your skin. Until recently, scientists believed that the signs of skin ageing – most noticeable as loss of skin tone and wrinkles – were largely due to the genes we inherited. But now dermatologists agree that up to 80 per cent of ageing is due to sun damage. Ultraviolet (UVA and UVB) rays in daylight cause damage to the structure of skin cells and trigger the increase of harmful

free radicals, harming the connective tissues that keep our skin firm. Other harmful ageing factors include a poor diet, dehydration, smoking, stress and alcohol.

sunscreens and skin health

In addition to rapid ageing, it is thought that severe sun damage causes the DNA destruction that leads to skin cancer. Even in mild, damp climates, the UVA rays that cause the most damage are present in large enough quantities to harm you during daylight hours. Wearing sunscreen with a sun-protection factor (SPF) of 15 on your face every day, even in winter, will help to prevent these risks. Many moisturisers now offer built-in SPF 15 protection, so look out for these skin protectors. And in summer, if you exercise outside, remember that all-over sunscreen is only part of your sun-protection plan. Wear a hat during the hottest part of the day, between 10am and 3pm, and cover up – long-sleeved tops and trousers will shield your body.

skin foods that work

Your skin relies on several vitamins to thrive. Most importantly, you should include plenty of vitamin C in your diet. The spongy, middle layer of your skin – the dermis – needs vitamin C to manufacture collagen, which keeps the skin smooth and wrinkle-free. It is thought that even a slight vitamin C deficiency may lower collagen production, so make sure that you eat five portions of fruit and vegetables daily (see pages 20–1). Other skin vitamins include vitamin E, which works with vitamin C, and is

---

THE BENEFITS OF SKIN PROTECTION

- Reduces the risk of cancer

- Reduces the signs of ageing by up to 80 per cent

- Better skin tone and flexibility

- Skin has fewer blemishes and looks radiant

---

found in oats and nuts. B vitamins, present in yeast, will also help. Calcium is key to skin maturity: you can find it in semi-skimmed milk and dairy products. A good daily multi-vitamin will contain the zinc and selenium you need for healthy skin cell growth and protection.

skin and moisturising

No matter how oily your skin is naturally, the drying effects of central heating and pollution can take their toll. And if you drink alcohol, this will dehydrate your skin further. The signs of dry skin include rough or reddened patches on the body, a dull look, and lines that are starting to look deeper. Even if you don't need a daily moisturiser, drinking eight glasses of water (up to 2 litres) daily will help your skin to maintain its natural elasticity and glow.

POST-WORKOUT AROMA MOISTURISER

Use this soothing oil to wind down after an exercise session, or simply make it a night-time treat once a week. To lock in maximum moisture, apply after a bath or shower while the skin is still damp.

1. Mix 3 dessertspoons of sweet almond oil with 2 drops of lavender essential oil and 1 drop of neroli (orange blossom) essential oil in a saucer.

2. Warm the oil in your hands by massaging a little of it between your palms.

3. Apply in long, feathery strokes to the arms and legs, moving in upward strokes.

4. Apply extra oil to the elbows and ankles, which can be particularly dry, and rub in well. Use this as an opportunity to soothe away any muscle stiffness.

record your progress

Fill in the blanks below to chart your success.

Measurements before the start of Week 06:	Measurements at the end of Week 06:
bust	bust
waist	waist
hips	hips
thighs	thighs
upper arms	upper arms

How many power walks did you do?

1   2   3   4

How many pedometer steps?

How many toning sessions did you do?

1   2   3   4

Rate your healthy eating this week

1   2   3   4   5   (1, poor and 5, excellent)

Rate your water intake this week

1   2   3   4   5   (1, poor and 5, excellent)

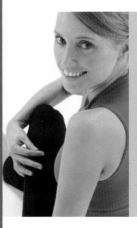

'Congratulations! You have completed the programme and are now a full-time member for life of the No-Gym Workout.'

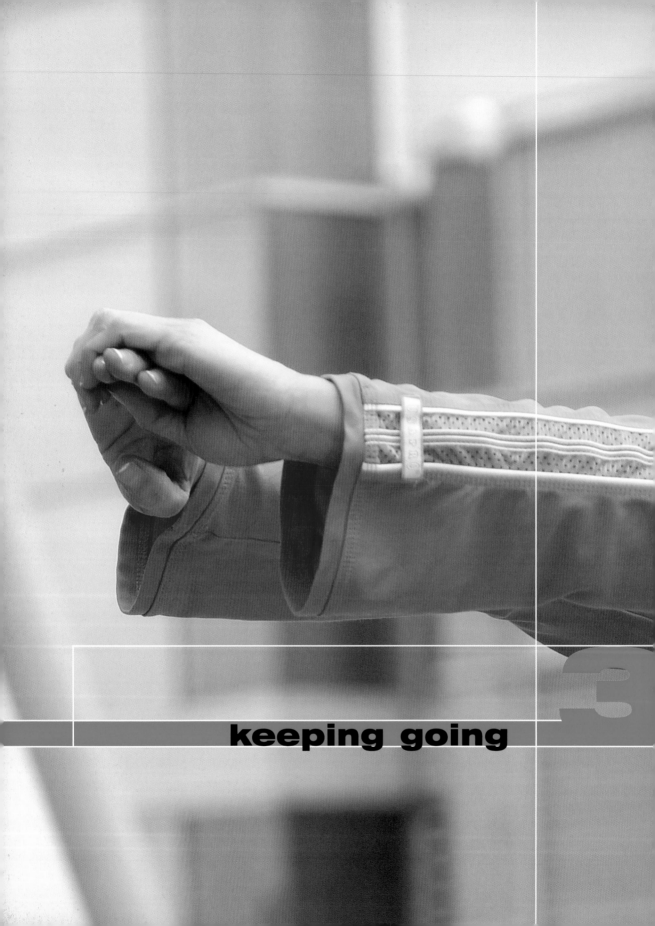

keeping going

3

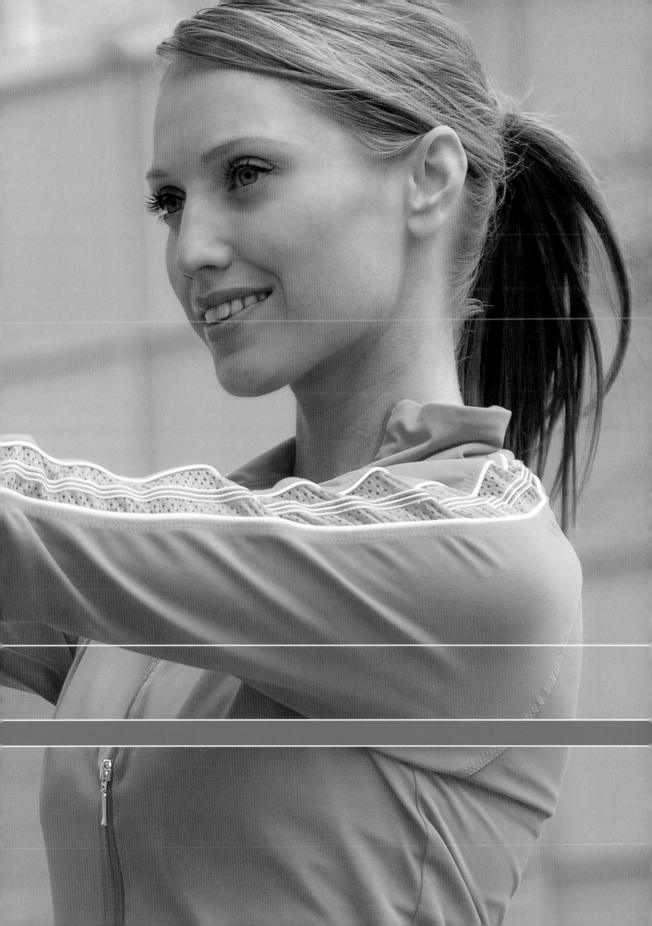

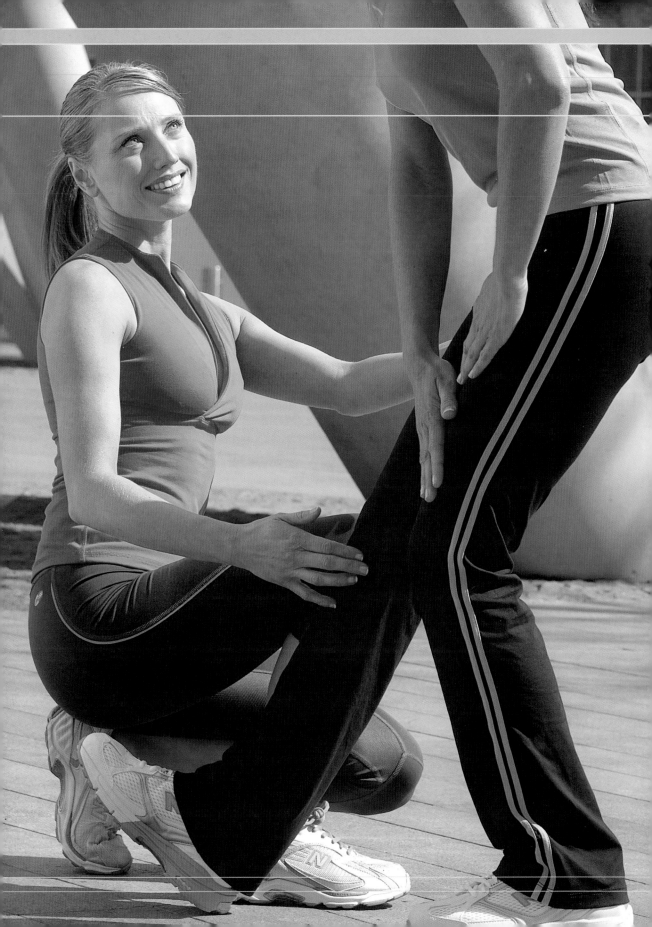

fine-tuning your shape

get to grips with your natural outline

Apple, pear or runner bean? Learn to love your figure whatever its natural shape is – then once you have completed the six-week programme keep it toned by creating a personal maintenance progamme designed especially for you. If you have had a baby recently, try my postnatal programme to get you back into the swing of exercising before you embark on the No-Gym Workout.

what's your body shape?
apple, pear or runner bean?

Women's bodies vary enormously and come in every size and shape. Size, shape and self-esteem seem to go hand in hand – we are subtly aware of other women's shapes on the train, at work, in the queue at the cashpoint, and constantly compare them to our own. What's important, however, is recognising and accepting our inherent shape, then toning to target problem areas.

You can't alter your fundamental body shape, but you can hone the wobbly bits and feel better about your body all round. Our case study Trea (see page 114) is a natural apple shape, holding her weight around her waist and stomach, yet she managed to lose 20cm (8in) from her waist measurement after six weeks on the programme – which proves that you can make significant improvements to your silhouette. Whatever body blueprint you were born with, you can exercise to enhance your shape at any stage of your life.

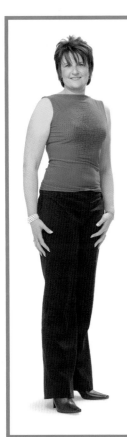

EACH SHAPE HAS ITS ADVANTAGES

My pear-shaped friend never stops asking me, 'Does my bum look big in this?' yet she forgets that she has the most amazing abs and tiny waist. Apple-shaped Trea (left), however, has naturally slim hips and legs and a small bottom. Runner beans, who berate their flat chests, are admired for their tall elegance and the fact that they look good in anything – whereas the pear must beware bottom-hugging skirts and jeans, and the apple needs floaty tops and tight trousers to play up slim legs and hide a midriff.

apple, pear and runner bean – the three body types

Here's how I keep it simple. Consider these three archetypal shapes: apple, pear and runner bean. Most women tend towards one of these shapes, although not exclusively. One way to ascertain which you are, if you're not already aware, is to ask yourself which areas of your body are most difficult to spot-reduce – tell-tale areas include the backs of the arms, cellulite on the thighs and bottom (pear), a chubby tummy and waist (apple) or, for the runner bean, a lack of curves. The idea of these three body types was put forward by American psychologist William Sheldon (1898–1977).

Mesomorph or apple: carry weight in the middle – waist and stomach, average to large bust
Metabolic rate: average

Endomorph or pear: slim waisted, sometimes a flat stomach, large bottom and thighs, bigger thighs than bust
Metabolic rate: average

Ectomorph or runner bean: straight up and down, small/flat chested, long arms and legs
Metabolic rate: high

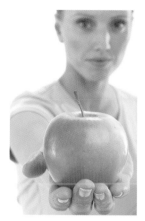

the apple circuit

These five exercises (see below) from the programme are ideal for apple shapes because the focus is on the abdominals. As apples tend to be heavier around the middle, gaining fat around the waist and stomach, these three middle-body exercises work deeply into the abdominal muscles and draw in the waist. You can also work your abs by keeping them drawn in tight when practising the upper- and lower-body exercises, the box press and gluteal circle.

A good exercise to try if you are apple-shaped is to place a belt or piece of string around your waist, pull your abs in tight then fasten the belt or tie the string. Now continue with your daily routine remembering to hold your abs in. Each time you forget and relax them you will be reminded by the tug on your belt or piece of string. Doing this exercise enhances your core strength, working on your transversus abdominis muscles while also strengthening your lower back.

power walking for apples I recommend using hand weights while you power walk (see page 36) and walk at a good fast pace – doing this will really work your oblique muscles, which draw in the waist. Remember to pull in your stomach whenever you walk. Halfway through your walk, put down the weights and do the standing oblique twist exercise (see pages 62–3), so adding toning to your power walk.

LUCY'S TUMMY TIP

Buy a pack of adhesive notes and write yourself a memo: 'Pull in my stomach and count to 10.' Put them wherever you spend time – on your desk at home or work, by the kettle in the kitchen, by the bathroom mirror. Every time you see your note, follow the instructions – and pull in your tummy. This activates your abdominals and gets you used to working these important muscles more regularly, not just when you follow the No-Gym abdominal exercises.

EXERCISES FOR APPLES

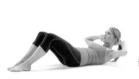

Abdominal crunch (from week 01: see pages 50–1)

Seated twist (from week 04: see pages 86–7)

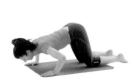

Box press (from week 01: see pages 48–9)

Abdominal roll (from week 05: see pages 98–9)

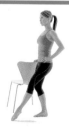

Gluteal circle (from week 05: see pages 100–1)

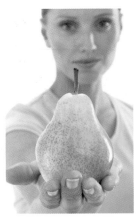

the pear circuit

Pears carry more weight around their hips, thighs, bottom and backs of the upper arms, although they tend to have fairly toned midriffs. These exercises from the programme (see below) focus mainly on the hips, bottom and legs, working all the major muscle groups. The abdominal exercise targets all the abdominal muscles, and the press-up is great for upper-body strength and for revving up the metabolic rate. The result of doing a combination of all three lower-body exercises is the equivalent of a non-surgical buttock lift.

power walking for pears Power walking up a slight incline is good for pear shapes as this really works the legs and buttocks harder than walking on even ground, but if you don't have a convenient hill outside your front door, just try the following interval training for extra toning power:

1 Begin power walking at a brisk pace.
2 Now walk faster and squeeze your bottom tight: hold the squeeze for 10 seconds, then release, and return to your previous pace. Draw your belly button tight to your spine to tone your abs as well as your bottom.
3 Repeat at intervals throughout your walk.

A variation on this style of interval training is to lengthen your stride for 10 paces at a time – striding out as if you're stepping over a puddle. This deeply tones your bottom as you extend your legs back.

LUCY'S BOTTOM-LIFTING TIP

Every time you go up the stairs from now on take them two steps at a time, avoiding using the hand rail, to give your bottom extra tone as a result of the deeper, wider movement. Take the stairs instead of the lift in shoping centres or at work – again going up two steps at a time. And if you have a spare few minutes at home – waiting for the kettle to boil, for example – run up and down the stairs a few extra times.

EXERCISES FOR PEARS

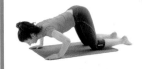

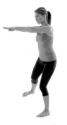

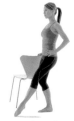

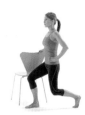

| Box press (from week 01: see pages 48–9) | Abdominal roll (from week 05: see pages 98–9) | Squat and lift (from week 04: see pages 88–9) | Gluteal circle (from week 05: see pages 100–1) | Lunge and kick (from week 01: see pages 52–3) |

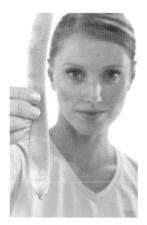

the runner bean circuit

Runner beans may look athletic, with a long torso and limbs, but looks can be deceiving. My tall, slim runner-bean friend looks svelte in jeans and a black roll neck jumper, but on the beach last summer she peeled off to reveal shorts and a bikini top – and I couldn't believe how flabby she was. As a size 8–10, she certainly was not overweight, but she had so little muscle tone it became obvious that her clothes held her in and gave her much-needed shape. Without them, she looked almost formless. Of course, this doesn't apply to all those who are long and lean, but it can be a common problem if you don't exercise regularly, and aim to build strength and muscle tone.

These exercises focus on increasing strength-enhancing posture, building strength and improving flexibility. The wide-leg squat boosts flexibility in the legs, the hamstring kick encourages good body posture, and the upper-body exercise opens up the chest and increases the range of movement. The abdominal exercises include the abdominal crunch (see pages 50–1), plus an ab crunch on the stability ball, which will help you to build more strength. When you become adept at working on the ball, go for this super-advanced pose: sit on the ball, pull in your stomach and slowly lift one foot an inch or so off the floor, and hold.

power walking for runner beans Do your regular power walks, but with weights to build strength in your arms. Walk to improve your posture: try interval walking, with your shoulders pulled back and tummy in for a few minutes, then release and repeat.

LUCY'S POSTURE TIP

On adhesive notes, write the words 'ice cube'.

Put the notes wherever you're likely to see them often, then programme yourself to imagine that whenever you see 'ice cube' you'll feel that an ice cube has just been dropped down your back. Do this, and you'll instantly squeeze your shoulders together and sit or stand straight.

EXERCISES FOR RUNNER BEANS

Seated row
(from week 04:
see pages 84–5)

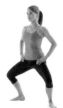

Wide-leg squat
(from week 02:
see pages 64–5)

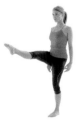

Hamstring kicks
(from week 03:
see pages 76–7)

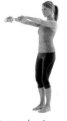

Lateral raise
(from week 06:
see pages 108–9)

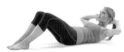

Abdominal crunch (from week 01: see pages 50–1) with stability ball.
(If you do not have a ball, do the plank, from week 06, pages 110–11)

postnatal workout
a new shape

Getting into shape after having a baby need not be a struggle, even when time for yourself and sleep are limited. Practise these exercises three times a week – there are only six to master – and you'll soon see results as you grow stronger and firmer. You can even work with your baby for two of the exercises (see pages 129 and 130) and enjoy maintaining eye contact throughout the movements.

The postnatal exercises in this section will benefit your mind and body, promoting better posture, less muscle tension, more relaxation and, above all, abdominal muscle tone. The leg stretch, thigh squeeze and pelvic tilt (see pages 128, 131, 133) are designed to power up the rectus abdominis – a pair of muscles located on each side of the abdomen. During pregnancy, these muscles separate to allow expansion as the baby grows, and the linea alba, the connective band of muscle that runs down the front of the abdomen, expands (see below). By practising these stomach exercises you'll strengthen the rectus abdominis and help to close the separation gap.

It's also vital to tone the pelvic floor muscles – the sling of muscles that supports the urethra, vagina and rectum – which are weakened during pregnancy. The thigh squeeze does this, encouraging any tears in the muscle fibres to heal.

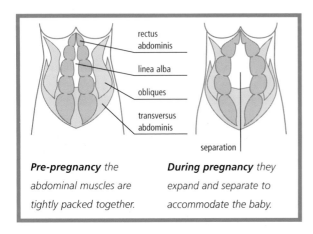

rectus abdominis

linea alba

obliques

transversus abdominis

separation

Pre-pregnancy *the abdominal muscles are tightly packed together.*

During pregnancy *they expand and separate to accommodate the baby.*

taking care

As with any exercise programme, you must ask your doctor for advice before beginning postnatal exercises. Only embark on the postnatal exercises here after you've had your six-week checkup and your doctor has confirmed that everything is fine. If any movement causes you the slightest pain or discomfort, stop immediately.

When you practise the postnatal exercises, work very slowly. Really focus on keeping your abdominal muscles pulled in. Also, it's vital that you don't overstretch. Before childbirth, the body releases a hormone called relaxin, which softens the pelvic bones. Relaxin can stay in the body for up to five or six months after your baby is born, which means it can be easy to overstretch muscles and cause injury. This is why the exercises in this section have relatively restricted movement, and don't involve freer moves such as kicks.

Also, don't overdo your workouts. A 10-minute session every other day will benefit you more than an hour's weekly guilt session, during which you're more likely to over-extend your body in a bid to catch up on lost time.

moving on to the six-week programme

Have a checkup with your doctor before beginning the six-week programme or any new fitness programme. Show your doctor the exercises in this book so he or she can see exactly what you might do.

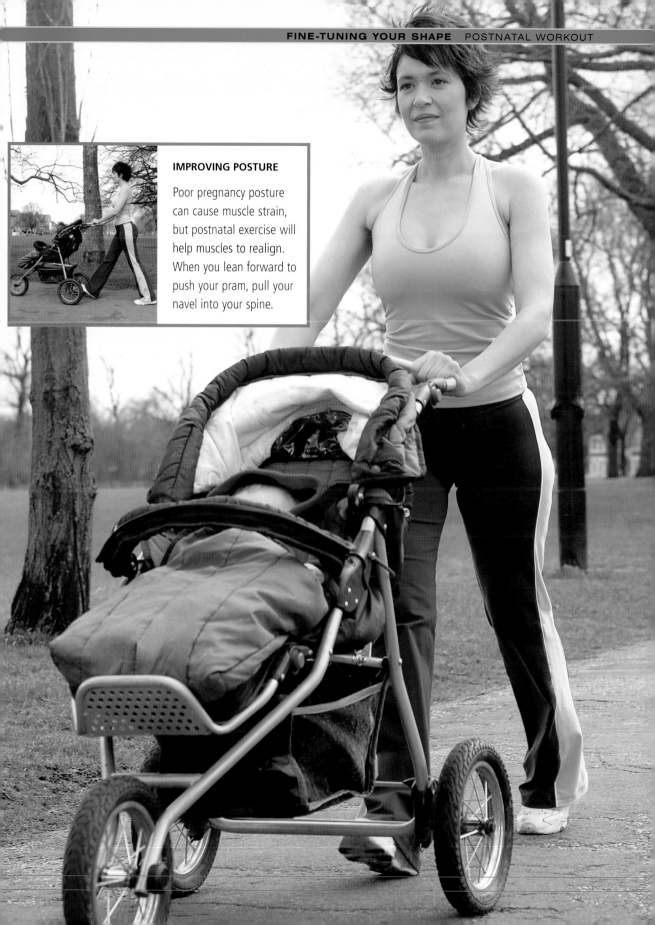

IMPROVING POSTURE

Poor pregnancy posture can cause muscle strain, but postnatal exercise will help muscles to realign. When you lean forward to push your pram, pull your navel into your spine.

postnatal workout
leg stretch

In the leg stretch, your stomach gets an intense workout. The transversus abdominis muscles of the stomach work hard to stabilise your lower body as you extend and retract one leg. It's a key move for boosting core stability.

WHAT DOES IT DO?

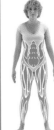

Draws in and strengthens the transversus abdominis muscles of the stomach.

calories burned	2
weekly calories	6

1

Keep your palms facing up to stop you pushing your weight through your hands

2

Tighten your abdominals to stabilise your hips as your legs move

the exercise

1 Lie on your back with your knees raised and your arms by your sides. Keep your palms facing upwards.

2 Breathe in then exhale as you pull your belly button to your spine and straighten one leg, sliding it along the floor.

3 Breathe in and exhale as you slide the leg back to a bending position.

repeat 12–20x

what to avoid

Don't let your back arch.

Don't forget to pull your belly button in to your spine.

kiss the baby

This box press trains the abdominal muscles and tones all the major muscles of the upper body, helping you to regain definition. You can work with your baby during this exercise, keeping eye contact and aiming for a kiss each time as you lower into the press-up.

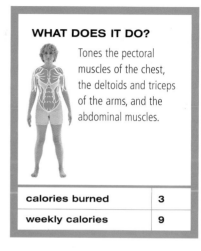

WHAT DOES IT DO?

Tones the pectoral muscles of the chest, the deltoids and triceps of the arms, and the abdominal muscles.

calories burned	3
weekly calories	9

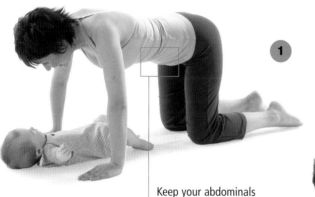

Keep your abdominals pulled in tight as you lower towards your baby

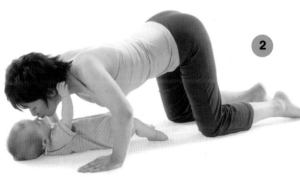

the exercise

1 Kneel on the floor with your knees directly under your hips. Your hands should be slightly wider than shoulder-width apart. Keep your fingers pointing forward, and check that your body weight is over your hands. Pull your tummy in tight, and keep your back flat. Imagine a straight line from your hips to your head keeping your body in alignment.

2 Breathe out as you lower your body, bending your arms so that your elbows make a 90-degree angle with the floor. Inhale as you push back up, pulling your navel to your spine.

repeat 12–20x

what to avoid

Avoid letting your back arch, relaxing the abdominal muscles so that your stomach sags. Keep the abdominal muscles taut for balance and to support your upper body as you move.

baby raises

This calf-raise exercise tones your lower legs and abdominals, and helps to improve your posture. Holding your baby, you'll tone your arms, and enjoy making eye contact as you move together.

WHAT DOES IT DO?

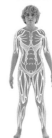

Tones the deepest abdominal muscles, along with the biceps and triceps of the arms and the calf muscles. Improves posture.

calories burned	4
weekly calories	12

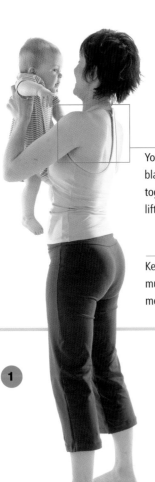

Your shoulder blades pull together as you lift your baby

Keep your abdominal muscles pulled in as you move onto your toes

1

2

the exercise

1 Stand with your feet hip-width apart. Pay attention to your posture, keeping your shoulders back and down.

2 Rise onto your tiptoes, and pull your navel into your spine. Hold for two seconds, then lower, returning to the starting position.

repeat 12–20x

what to avoid

Don't lock out your knees.

Don't arch your back – keep it straight and shoulders down.

thigh squeeze

The thigh squeeze strengthens your pelvic floor muscles, and is brilliant for toning your inner thighs without causing any impact to your joints. You'll need a pillow or cushion for this exercise.

WHAT DOES IT DO?

Works the pelvic floor muscles and adductor muscles of the inner thighs.

calories burned	2
weekly calories	6

Squeeze your thighs as tightly as you can

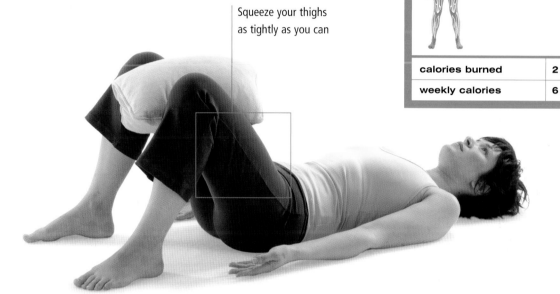

the exercise

1 Lie on the floor with your knees up. Place a pillow or cushion between your knees. Place your arms by your sides, with your palms facing upwards.

2 Breathe in, then, as you exhale, press your knees together. Hold for two seconds, then release. Focus on keeping your upper body relaxed as your lower body works hard.

repeat 12–20x

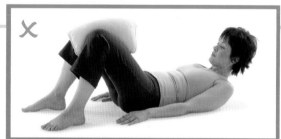

what to avoid

Don't lift your back off the floor or use your hands to take the pressure off the squeeze. This may strain your back, and it reduces the intensity of the squeeze.

chest press

Great for toning the chest and arms, this move also strengthens the abdominals. Working on the floor, rather than standing, prevents overstretching. You'll need small hand weights or water bottles.

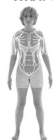
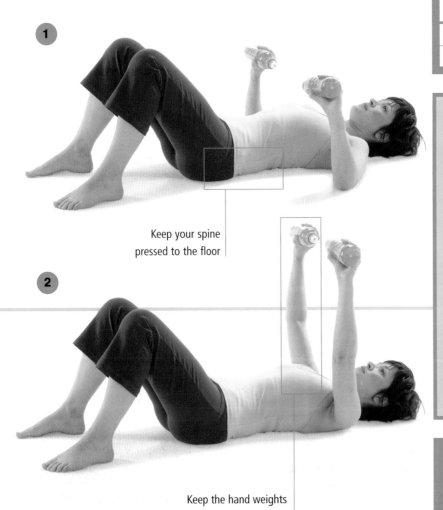

1

Keep your spine pressed to the floor

2

Keep the hand weights in line with your chest

the exercise

1 Lie on the floor with your knees up. Take hold of your weights, with your elbows out to the sides.

2 Breathe in then breathe out, pulling your navel in to your spine and extending your arms above your shoulders. Hold for two seconds, breathe in and pull your navel in again as you exhale and lower your arms back down into the starting position.

repeat 12–20x

what to avoid

Don't let your arms drop over your head – keep them extended above your shoulders.

pelvic tilt

This precise movement has amazing benefits: it draws in the expanded abdominal muscles, builds strength in the lower back, and helps to realign the spine following poor posture during pregnancy.

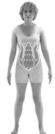

WHAT DOES IT DO?

Shortens the long rectus abdominis muscle, which is lengthened during pregnancy, and strengthens the transversus abdominis muscles of the stomach.

calories burned	2
weekly calories	6

Keep the tilt slow and controlled

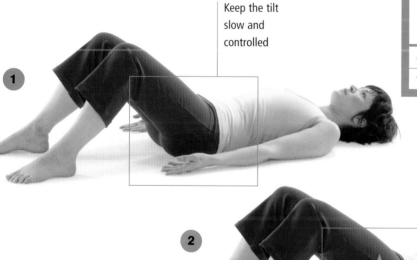

1

As you tilt, pull up and in

2

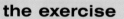

the exercise

1 Lie on the floor with your knees bent and your arms relaxed by your sides. Check that your spine is in 'neutral' – in a line with your hips and shoulders, and not arched.

2 Breathe in, then exhale gently as you pull your naval towards your spine and tilt your pelvis so the pubic bone lifts and your lower back presses into the floor. Hold for two seconds and release, returning to the starting position.

repeat 12–20x

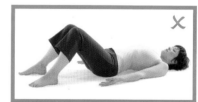

what to avoid

Don't arch your back – it should move only from the neutral position to the tilted position.

beyond six weeks
continuing your workout

After you've completed the No-Gym Workout, here's how to continue with the regime and adapt the exercises to suit your needs. Whether you want to look your best for a long-awaited holiday or for a special celebration, your confidence will double when you know you're working your body in the right way to get results – and all without having the added pressure of getting to a gym when you're extra busy.

Keeping active is the first step towards maintaining your shape and losing weight. Build as much exercise into your daily routine as you can. Frequent short walks to the shops add up to a good power walk, so don't feel guilty if you can't always fit in a full 20- or 30-minute stretch. Walk rather than drive for all your short daily trips to keep the momentum up, and whenever you can, exercise early in the day. This not only gets you feeling in control of your day, but it also revs up your metabolism so you burn off more calories before lunch.

step up the programme

If you have a special event to prepare for, you can step up the exercise programme to include two exercises for the upper, middle or lower body. Look through the programme and choose a total of three extra exercises, so you'll be doing six exercises three times a week instead of three

---

WEDDING BOOT CAMP

If you are toning up because you're getting married, I advise you to focus very much on the exercises for the middle body to get you feeling comfortable in your dress, and on training the upper body so you'll feel super-confident showing your arms. Middle- and upper-body exercises will also improve your posture and help you to walk tall.

---

exercises three times a week, effectively doubling your effort. This will get you speedy results, because the extra variation stops your body from hitting a plateau – when your muscles become used to what you're doing.

keep it varied

Keep to the same set of exercises for a maximum of four weeks, then vary the programme by choosing a different combination of upper-, middle- and lower-body exercises. The more variety you have, the more likely it is that you'll stay with your regime. Here's a mix-and-match example:

Weeks 01 to 03
- Abdominal crunch (week 01)
- Wide-leg squat (week 02)
- Overhead arm press (week 03)

Weeks 04 to 06
- Seated twist (week 04)
- Criss-cross arms (week 05)
- The bridge (week 06)

To keep your power walks varied, use the power walking programme (see page 37). Note when to use hand weights and when to step up the intensity.

boost the burn

A great option is to work through the six-week programme again from the beginning, this time opting to boost the burn. If you haven't tackled these moves yet, you'll feel challenged and burn even more calories as you work out.

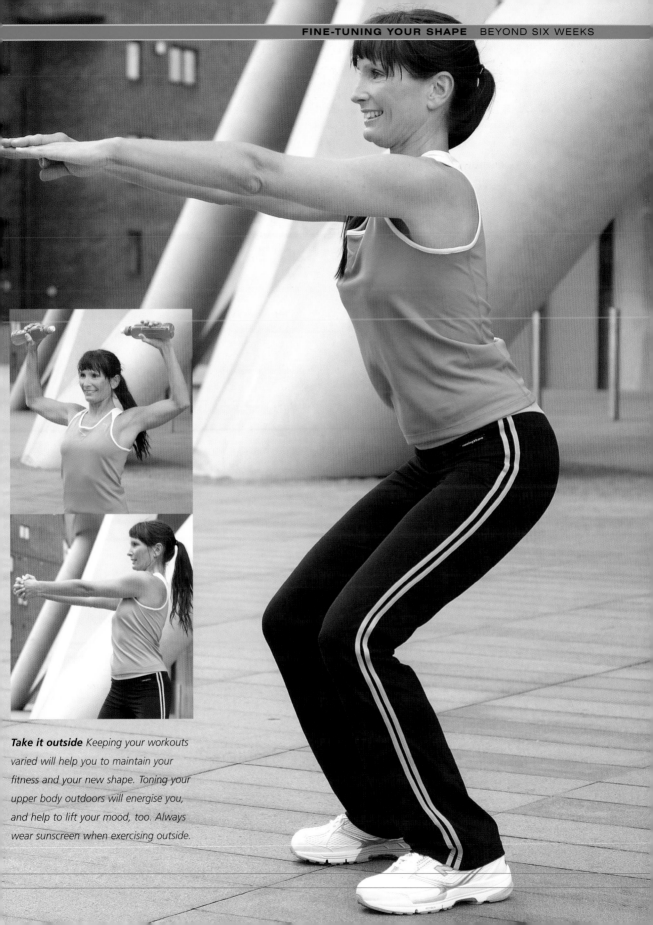

Take it outside Keeping your workouts varied will help you to maintain your fitness and your new shape. Toning your upper body outdoors will energise you, and help to lift your mood, too. Always wear sunscreen when exercising outside.

visual index
weeks 01 and 02

Here's an easy way to remind yourself of the entire six-week sequence at a glance. You may find it helpful to photocopy these pages and pin them up close to wherever you do your toning exercises.

O1
box press

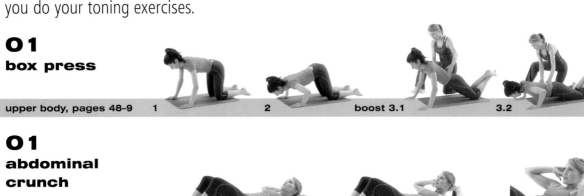

upper body, pages 48–9   1   2   boost 3.1   3.2

O1
abdominal crunch

middle body, pages 50–1   1   2   boost 3

O1
lunge and kick

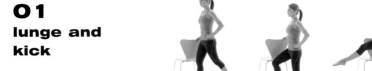

lower body, pages 52–3   1   2   3   boost 4   5

O2
elbow and bust press

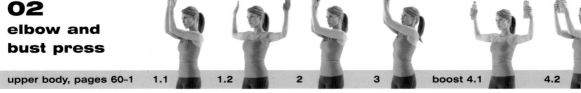

upper body, pages 60–1   1.1   1.2   2   3   boost 4.1   4.2

O2
standing oblique twist

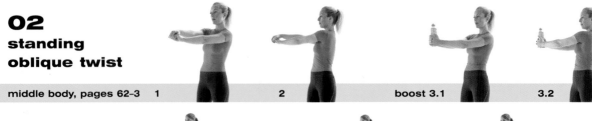

middle body, pages 62–3   1   2   boost 3.1   3.2

O2
wide-leg squat

lower body, pages 64–5   1   2   boost 3.1   3.2   4.1   4.2

weeks 03 and 04

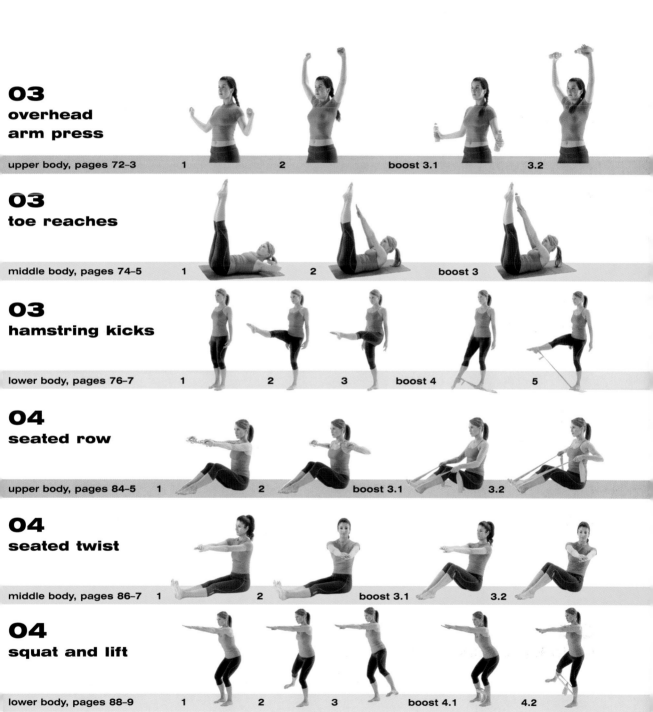

03
**overhead
arm press**

upper body, pages 72–3   1   2   boost 3.1   3.2

03
toe reaches

middle body, pages 74–5   1   2   boost 3

03
hamstring kicks

lower body, pages 76–7   1   2   3   boost 4   5

04
seated row

upper body, pages 84–5   1   2   boost 3.1   3.2

04
seated twist

middle body, pages 86–7   1   2   boost 3.1   3.2

04
squat and lift

lower body, pages 88–9   1   2   3   boost 4.1   4.2

weeks 05 and 06

05
criss-cross arms

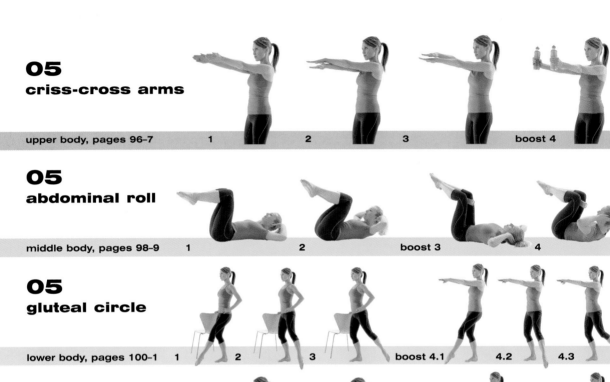

upper body, pages 96–7   1   2   3   boost 4

05
abdominal roll

middle body, pages 98–9   1   2   boost 3   4

05
gluteal circle

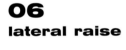

lower body, pages 100–1   1   2   3   boost 4.1   4.2   4.3

06
lateral raise

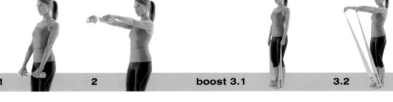

upper body, pages 108–9   1   2   boost 3.1   3.2

06
the plank

middle body, pages 110–11   1   2   boost 3

06
the bridge

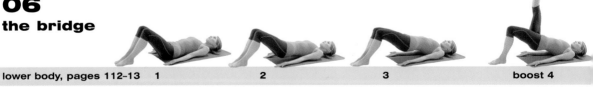

lower body, pages 112–13   1   2   3   boost 4

postnatal workout

As with the six-week sequences, here are mini-reminders of the postnatal routine. It's amazing to think that these six exercises are all you need to sculpt your shape into the figure you want in the months after you've had your baby.

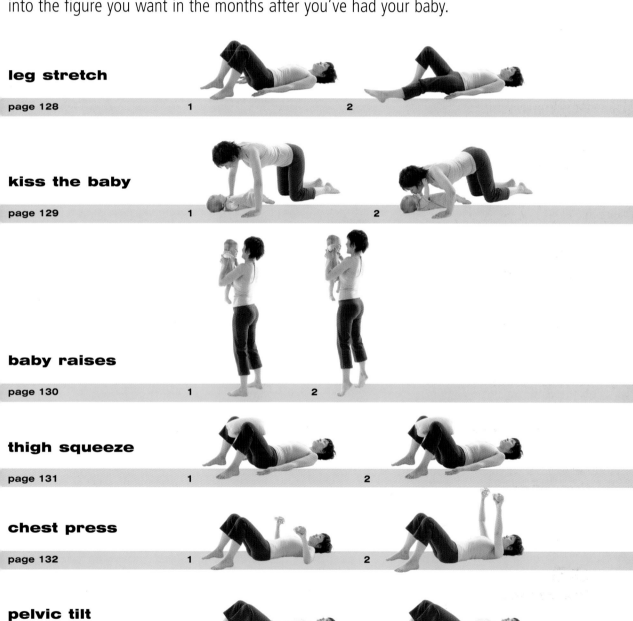

leg stretch
page 128   1   2

kiss the baby
page 129   1   2

baby raises
page 130   1   2

thigh squeeze
page 131   1   2

chest press
page 132   1   2

pelvic tilt
page 133   1   2

resources

sporting bodies

Department for Culture,
Media and Sport
www.culture.gov.uk

UK Sport
www.uksport.gov.uk
Working in partnership with sports
councils and other agencies to lead
UK sport to world-class success.

Sport England
www.sportengland.org
Working on the development of
sport in England. See also Sports
Councils for Northern Ireland, Wales
and Scotland.

Sports Council for Northern Ireland
www.sportni.net

Sports Council for Wales
www.sports-council-wales.co.uk

Sport Scotland
www.sportscotland.org.uk

health organisations

National Osteoporosis Society
www.nos.org.uk

British Heart Foundation
www.bhf.org.uk

British Thyroid Foundation
www.btf-thyroid.org

Diabetes UK
www.diabetes.org.uk

The British Menopause Society.
www.the-bms.org

Cancer Research UK Sunsmart
www.cancerresearchuk.org/sunsmart
Provides information about sun
protection and skin cancer.

British Wheel of Yoga
www.bwy.org.uk
Promotes yoga classes and workshops,
helping with breathing management.

food and nutrition

Women's Nutritional Advisory Service
www.naturalhealthas.com
Promotes healthier eating.

British Nutrition Foundation
www.nutrition.org.uk
Scientific and educational charity
providing advice and information
about nutrition.

British Dietetic Association
www.bda.uk.com
Advises on nutrition and health.

European Food Information Council
www.eufic.org
Guide to food safety and quality as
well as health and nutrition for a
healthy lifestyle.

Food Standards Agency
www.foodstandards.gov.uk
Independent government body
protecting consumer interests
in relation to food.

The Vegetarian Society
www.vegsoc.org
Offers advice on vegetarian
nutritional issues.

Weight Concern
www.weightconcern.org.uk
Charity working to tackle obesity as
well as helping people to improve
their health and feel good about
themselves, whatever their weight.

equipment suppliers

www.sweatybetty.com
Stockists of ladies' fitness clothing.

www.sheactive.co.uk
Stockists of ladies' fitness clothing.

www.girlsruntoo.co.uk
Stockists of ladies' fitness clothing.

www.ronhill.co.uk
Stockists of ladies' fitness clothing.

www.sweatshop.co.uk
Stockists of ladies' fitness clothing.

www.lessbounce.com
Stockists of a wide range of
sports bras.

www.simplysports.com
Stockists of a wide range of sports
equipment including hand weights,
resistance bands, pedometers, mats.

www.heartratemonitor.co.uk
Suppliers of a wide range of heart
rate monitors used to calculate
calorie burn.

sporting charities

www.raceforlife.org
Information about local 5km charity
walks for women raising money for
breast cancer.

www.ramblers.org.uk
For free organised walks.

overseas resources

Australia
The Australian Sport Commission
www.ausport.gov.au
Government body providing leadership
in all facets of sport.

Nutrition Australia
www.nutritionaustralia.org
Scientific nutrition information.

Health First
www.healthfirst.net.au
Provides easy access to health
information.

Health MG
www.healthmg.com.au
Suppliers of sports equipment
and services.

New Zealand
Sport and Recreation New Zealand
www.sparc.org.nz
Dedicated to getting New Zealanders
active, supporting elite athletes
as well as sport in local communities.

Millennium Institute of Sport
and Health
www.institutesporthealth.org.nz
Helping people of all ages and levels
to become fitter and healthier.

NZ Nutrition Foundation
www.foodworks.co.nz/
nutritionfoundation
Nutrition education, research,
promotion and evaluation.

Polar
www.polarheart.co.nz
Suppliers of heart rate monitors.

South Africa
Sports and Recreation South Africa
www.srsa.gov.za
National department for sports
and recreation.

SA HealthInfo
www.sahealthinfo.org
Government-initiated project providing
comprehensive health information.

Nutrition Information Centre,
University of Stellenbosch
webhost.sun.ac.za/nicus
Independent source of nutrition
information.

index

acknowledgments

Models: Amaya Alvarez, Rachel Black, Corinne and Alex Roberts, Kelly Suleman, Dominique Swinton-Bland, Tracey Young, Natalie Gartshore, Trea Stacey, Emma Johnson, Ella Upton, Jessica Coombes, Jess Sproule, Karen Phillipson

Photo credits: Page 22 - bl - Maren Caruso; br - Jim Franco; page 39 - tr - Berit Myrekrok/Digital Vision/Getty
Medical advisor: Dr Tom Smith
Nutritionist: Sue Baic
Photographer's assistants: Sarah Bailey, Angus Northover and Charlotte Brown
Hair and makeup: Maza White (hair stylist and makeup), Jackie Dixon from SeanHanna (case studies' hair stylist)
Models' clothes: Sweaty Betty, She-Active and Linda Clarke

Rodale thanks
Extra special thanks to Mike Prior, for shooting such fantastic photos, to all the wonderful case studies for participating in The No-Gym Workout and for being such good sports, to Sweaty Betty, She-Active and Linda Clarke for so generously lending us the models' clothes and shoes; to www.heartratemonitor.co.uk for the loan of the watches that enabled us to calculate the calories burned for the exercises, to www.simplysports. com who kindly supplied us with sports equipment; to Dr Tom Smith and nutritionist Sue Baic for their assistance and advice; and finally, thanks to Anne Newman for proofreading and Hilary Bird for the index.

From the author
A special thanks to Liz Coghill and Anne Lawrance at Rodale for having such vision and making this happen. Thanks also to my agent Borra Garson and all at Deborah McKenna Ltd for helping me on this journey; to Hannah Moore for having an eye for style and making it all look so fantastic; to Maza White who is a truly amazing makeup artist and for making us all laugh lots; to Mike Prior, whose photography is great – just like his sense of humour – and his lovely assistants. Special thanks to Liz Dean and Angela Baynham for their amazing skills and ability to literally take the words right out of my mouth.

A very big thanks to all my wonderful clients who have given me support and encouragement; to all the case studies for their time and commitment – Ella, Karen, Trea, Jessie, Emma and my beautiful sister Jessica; to Simon for making me so determined to make this happen; to Dommie and Tracey for modelling and looking great.

Love and thanks to all of my family and friends, especially to my wonderful Mum and Dad who have been my inspiration, and to Jess, Johnny, Harriet, Tom, Amelia and Keith for all their support.

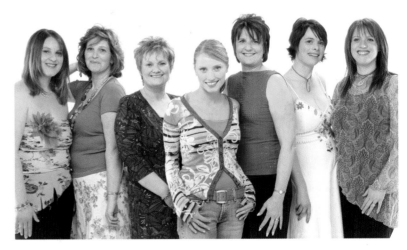